THE BEST OF
HEALTHY LIVING

LORI BROTHERS

ACKNOWLEDGEMENTS

I wish to thank all of the enthusiastic, dedicated readers of my weekly, "Healthy Living," column, you inspire me to inspire you; the New Castle News publication, and especially Dan Irwin and Jessica Schelenberger, for their collaboration and support; Jameson Health System, New Castle, Pennsylvania, which has provided me an avenue to share my passion for healthy living concepts and lifestyle education.

I would like to express my deepest respect and appreciation for Dr. Dean Ornish, and The Dean Ornish Program For Reversing Heart Disease, a foundational research project which has proven clinically that healthy lifestyle is medicine with the power to reverse disease in the human body; and all of the patients and participants of on-going "Ornish living" who prove daily the potent medicine of empowered choice.

I appreciate the talents and collaboration of my colleague and friend, Lisa Lombardo, who has been so instrumental in launching "Healthy Living," and the completion of this project, including her expertise in cover design.

Most importantly, I thank my children, Corinne and Claire Brothers, who are my constant inspiration, and my proof that focusing on inner and outer health shapes remarkable people and develops the capacity for the most extraordinary living.

TABLE OF CONTENTS

I

II

Yoga: Developing Self-Awareness

Introduction

I invite you to make a resolution to look at what is unique and remarkable about the way you live your life. You already own these traits even though, sometimes, you may lose your appreciation for your authentic talents in the frenzy of everyday living. You probably aren't often invited to pay attention to the moments when you are living your best. Look for traits that example your talents and purpose.

Efficiency is very admirable, such as the habit of list-making. Some people don't make lists at all. They are worse off than those of us who try to keep order in our lives. Making order may be one of your gifts.

If you see someone looking a little disheveled, please be kind. They are probably not a list maker and need your support. Open the door for them. Flash them an understanding smile. Compassion is remarkable. Then, with list in hand, thank God that you've made a little order.

Consistency also ranks as a noteworthy pattern. Repeated right action that delivers the results you intended is truly remarkable in a world that is moving fast. Are you creating the patterns that support your happiness, health and well-being? Regular routines create good habits. The definition of a habit is "a usual way of behaving; something that a person does often in a regular and repeated way," according to Merriam-Webster. Therefore, good habits rank as remarkable.

A remarkable mind-set is also the key to creating new habits or developing the ones that bring out your best. Let go of judgment and guilt. They shadow the remarkable. Be willing to objectively observe your attitudes and thought patterns. Yank out those underwhelming "mind weeds" that set you up for unremarkable living. When it comes to creating good habits don't set yourself up for failure by attempting weak or rigid attitudes, such as taking the stance of "always" or "never." This will lead to self-sabotage.

It is far more effective to develop positive trending in both thought and action. Pay attention to your trends when you are at your best. You'll know it by the remarkable results. Keep your sights on what you usually do well, and do more of that.

Dedicate this year, starting right now, to finding the remarkable in yourself. What makes you the best you? This may take some serious reflection. Tune-in to be your best by answering these questions:

- What are your tendencies for utilizing spare time?
- How do you interact with your family and friends when you are contributing or sharing?
- What are your talents when engaged in purposed work or activities?
- What is your eating style?
- What food choices contribute to your health goals?

- Who are your role models?
- Do you follow those good examples?
- Are you a good example for others?
- What habits block my best and my ability to grow?
- What habits can I practice to activate the best that I can contribute?

The short reads in this book are meant to trigger your curiosity. Become curious about how you can better understand best of your personal purpose and talents. It is the truly remarkable human who takes the time to know and live the answers to the questions above, and other personally compelling questions.

I invite you to decide that now is the time to appreciate, further develop, and begin to reveal your remarkable you. Be willing to shine.

Learn From the Fated Frog

You may have heard of the experiment where a frog is put into a pan of cool water and watched as, over time, the temperature of the water is increased. The frog does not seem to notice the increasing temperature as it acclimates slowly to the rising temperature. It is gruesome to know that the frog will allow itself to boil to death.

Yet research compares this acclimation process to what many Americans do with their diets as they increase in the amounts of sugar, fat and salt in their food consumption. The result of unconscious choice-making creeps up over time and can lure us into the "pleasure trap." Just as the sensory capabilities of the frog failed to adequately warn him to survive, it is very easy to lose the ability to discern how much salt, sugar and fat you are taking in, relying only on what you become accustomed to eating based on overly sensitized taste buds.

Taste buds are sensory nerves and can easily lock onto high levels of stimulation. The sense of taste can be trained to seek and recognize artificially high levels of added flavors, steering us as eaters into more and more exaggerated taste experiences. Eating without the awareness of how often you choose these foods can have dangerous consequences. This makes less stimulating, health-promoting foods less appealing.

Without balanced choice making, you can sabotage your flavor pallet and threaten your health.

In all of the years that I have seen many people successfully choose to retrain their taste buds, learn to eat new flavors and textures, and choose new habits – I still always hold a concern for the many who may not be fully aware that they are setting themselves up for premature death. Unnecessary risk factors such as diabetes, high blood pressure and high cholesterol, stir a preamble to more serious disease including heart attacks and strokes, because they have fallen into the pleasure trap.

The brain also has a role in choosing over-stimulating foods. A chemical called Dopamine affects our brain processes, controlling our movement, emotional response, and ability to experience pleasure and pain. "Dopamine is the chemical that mediates pleasure in the brain. It is released during pleasurable situations and stimulates one to seek out the pleasurable activity or occupation. This means food, sex, and so many several drugs of abuse are also stimulants of dopamine release in the brain," said Dr. Ananya Mandal, MD, in her article posted on www.news-medical.net.

Once these patterns are established and associated with pleasure but often void of nourishment, it becomes more difficult to eat mindfully without perceiving that you are giving up pleasure for your health. Once you desensitize your taste buds to over-stimulation, you will learn to enjoy the natural flavors of foods, and find pleasure in eating well.

Eating well leads to feeling well. Feeling the positive sensation of amplified physical energy levels, and the elimination of pain as inflammation recedes from a body that has lower in-puts of fat, salt and sugar, is worth re-training the tongue. Become willing to learn to value natural fresh foods over processed foods. My hope is that you hop into action to reprogram your taste buds and redefine pleasure to mean feeling great.

Make the decision not to become the fated frog. Pay close attention to when you are choosing over-salted or sugary drinks and high-fat foods and snacks too often. The more you acclimate yourself to these sensations and flavors, the more you are hooked by the pleasure trap, the more you slowly enter the boiling water of our times, and the harder it is to eat more natural tasting foods.

Be the Difference

"Health is a state of complete physical, mental and social well-being, and not merely the absence of disease or infirmity," was a statement issued by the World Health Organization in 1948.

During that year, Harry Truman was named Time Magazine's "Man of the Year." The quote of the year was, "And now it's time for a really big show" (pronounced "shoe"), by Ed Sullivan.

The Ford F-series truck was introduced. Scrabble (the board game) was invented, and was the most popular Christmas present that year. Bar codes were also invented this same year. (Aha, there's the glitch that made the whole culture come unglued.)

Think about how our culture has changed since then. Women have become much more anchored in the work force, eating fast foods for many is now a way of living, and sedentary lifestyle is also on the rise. I won't go so far to say we are all living fast and tired...but doesn't it sometimes feel that way?

Mark Twain observed, "The only way to keep your health is to eat what you don't want, drink what you don't like, and do what you'd druther not."

We're told "eat this, not that," on a regular basis, inundated with conflicting philosophies. So if you're paying attention you may have a side of guilt with those fries. If guilt doesn't get you, there's a chance your simmering health issues might.

Obesity trends among U.S. adults were studied over a 20-year period to reveal staggering results. The Center for Disease Control and Prevention defined obesity as approximately 30 pounds overweight.

In 1990, the adult U.S. population weighed-in with approximately a 10-14 percent obesity rate. In 1999, that figure rose to approximately 20-24 percent. By 2008 statistics showed that well over 29 percent of the U.S. population is obese. The figures vary from state to state. However, the statistics show the alarming increase, and the disease rates that correspond. Studies also indicate that there was a 600 percent increase in diabetes between 1950 and 1993. That is staggering.

Dr. Dean Ornish's book, *The Spectrum*, points out, "Our genes did not change during this period, only our diet and lifestyle changed."

So as we now download the next app onto our cell phones to help us keep track of our calories, or plot out our exercise routines, let's stop to remember a simpler time.

Maybe eating a healthy snack while playing a board game, after taking an evening walk is the answer. Wait a minute what year are we living in? Can we get the kids away from their wi-fi?

So back to the World Health Organization which named physical, mental and social well-being as the definition of health.

If we choose to focus on good habits and wise choices and we can lick much of the disease and infirmity that is so prevalent in our culture today.

Does that mean fast food is out the window? (Just a little fast food pun – for fun.) I think not. It's more about a shift in awareness.

Stephen Covey said, "The key is not to prioritize what's on your schedule, but to schedule your priorities."

So instead of contending with conflicting food advice, consider the maxim "eat more of this, less of that." Also, schedule time for a walk, social connection and getting enough rest. These have been proven priorities that steer away from disease and towards health.

Prioritizing can make you a part of a new trend in a new era. Because when we reflect on it, we have the opportunity to make the difference now that those in the future may be looking back on in 20 years. Be the difference. Our descendants will be proud…and hopefully healthier.

A Human Stick of Butter

There's a great line in the movie "Two Weeks Notice," a 2002 romantic comedy film starring Hugh Grant and Sandra Bullock, where a husband and wife are talking and the wife says, "Larry, your cholesterol is over 300...you're basically a solid." I can just imagine the guy standing there – a human stick of butter.

Funny. Yet, the chuckling may end if you have a cholesterol level over 200, the recommended guideline. Is your blood congealing as you read this? It is the reason why there is a guideline. Thick blood from high cholesterol and high triglycerides leads to higher risk of high blood pressure, stroke, coronary artery disease and heart attack. Do you know your numbers?

What is the purpose of cholesterol? All of your cells have this wax-like substance, cholesterol, produced by your liver, which is needed to help you digest foods, aide in the production of bile, create hormones, insulate nerve fibers and convert sunshine to Vitamin D.

So, with all of that important stuff going on, why the concern about having too much cholesterol in your blood stream? It is important to note that body produces its own cholesterol and stores what it does not use for these natural functions. Unfortunately, we can't just pour more cholesterol into our bodies and let it flow right back out. Remember, the body stores it.

Since cholesterol is also found in many of the foods we eat in our American cuisine, we are prone to put far more cholesterol in, resulting in growing numbers of increased disease-related processes. The thought of walking around with pudding-like blood in your veins may be a reason to look again at the foods you are eating. There are no visible signs of high cholesterol. Only a blood test can get you the information you need.

It is better to know where you stand when it comes to this very important issue. Depending on where you numbers fall can be the motivational factor to help you seek the help you need from your doctor and good education about lifestyle changes that can be life saving.

There are those who do not want this kind of education...ignorance is bliss. There are those of you who have some education and choose not to act on what you know. There are many more of you reading this that are committed to learning and applying what you learn. Even small changes can make a big impact.

If the culprits of animal fats are haunting your diet, and you are not the type to go vegetarian, then it is important to look at other areas where you can make a real improvement in your overall cholesterol readings. Choose leaner cuts of meat and increase your awareness regarding label reading to lower your intake of added saturated fats. If the label shows more than 5 grams of fat...put it back!

Triglycerides are another measure of how thick your blood is and the statistics suggest that if your total calories from carbohydrates -- anything that turns to sugar, i.e., white flour, white pasta and rice, added sweeteners -- exceeds 60 percent of your diet, you are at a high risk of elevated triglycerides. If you intake more that you burn, the sugar, which the body converts into glucose, ends up in the liver where it stores as triglycerides.

Choose to be smart with your choices about fats in your diet. The threat of morphing into a vat of shortening diminishes each time you pay attention to a label and limit your intake of saturated fats and heavy meats.

Become the Tortoise, Not the Bear

The threat of becoming "de-conditioned" hangs like the dark clouds of a Nor'easter over all of us who are about to head into winter in Western Pennsylvania. Research is showing that sitting around too long, even when you have a regular exercise routine, does damage to your body systems. The human body needs to move, and then move again. Regular intervals of movement jump start your body's systems and keep you charged – body and mind.

Certain mammals get the luxury of hibernating during the winter. Skunks and woodchucks do it. So do raccoons, chipmunks, hedgehogs, hamsters, bears and bats. However, for humans keeping movement in daily routine is the key to maintaining good health.

When it's icy, cold, snowing, and windy, there can be a fight for that parking space closest to the door in the store parking lot. Rarely do we purposely choose to park further from the door to get extra exercise in the winter, as we might during warmer seasons. My dog goes out the back door on her leash to do her business while I stand in the garage, protected from the winter elements. There's much less "walking the dog" in the winter.

When we're stuck inside due to blustery weather, we tend to eat more, sit more and snooze more. Therefore, if you don't make a mindful decision to move more while you are inside, there is a risk for substantial health decline. We must admit that because we often wear bulky, warm clothing we can deny problem areas that emerge. Out of sight, out of mind…as the saying goes. Meanwhile, hidden rolls and bulges under all those layers of clothes develop into the dreaded "winter pudge."

Sedentary lifestyle is responsible for an estimated $24 billion in direct medical spending (Americashealthranking.org). Increasing physical activity, especially from a complete absence of exercise, cannot only prevent numerous chronic diseases, it can also help to manage them. Approximately 2 million deaths per year are attributed to physical inactivity, prompting WHO (World Health Organization) to issue a warning that a sedentary lifestyle could very well be among the 10 leading causes of death and disability in the world.

You don't have to join a gym to get the kind of movement in your day you need to keep you away from the doctor and the ailments that come from lack of moving your body. Muscle tone, joints, and core strength can be maintained just by moving about 10 minutes, three times per day. I had the gift and pleasure of knowing a dear woman who lived to be 103 years old. She walked around her dining room table several times per day. She got it. She knew movement keeps the fire going, the mind strong, and the brain cobweb-free. I'm remembering wise Aunt Lilly. She had spunk.

How would you feel if you went to the doctor and he said he was treating you for lack of exercise? Mayo Clinic physiologist, Michael Joyner, M.D., has stated that lack of exercise should be treated as a medical condition. "When de-conditioned people try to exercise, they may tire quickly and experience dizziness or other discomfort, then give up trying to exercise and find the problem gets worse rather than better," Joyner says.

"If we were to medicalize it (exercise), we could then develop a way, just like we've done for addiction, cigarettes and other things, to give people treatments, and lifelong treatments, that focus on behavioral modifications and physical activity," says Joyner.

Visualize being the tortoise…slow and steady wins the winter race, instead of the bulky, slumbering bear in hibernation this winter. Just get up and move for 10-minute intervals. The evidence shows that if you establish a pattern of regular movement, you reap the significant health benefits that come from maintaining patterns of movement to combat the effects of sedentary de-conditioning during winter months, or in any season of your life that's got you sitting or laying down too long.

If It's Got Color, It's Got Health

There are a lot of numbers you are supposed to be aware of, in order to be clear about where you stand with your health, and to make your health goals. Do you know your numbers for your blood pressure, cholesterol, glucose and body mass index? Knowing these important numbers can help you identify what steps you need to take to reduce your risk for developing a chronic disease. You can contact your health care professional to establish a baseline, if you don't know your numbers, or if you're not current.

Now, let's also talk some interesting numbers that deliver great results directly to the cellular level of your body. There are over 150 phytochemicals in just one apple, which delivers a multitude of health benefits to humans. The saying, "an apple a day keeps the doctor away," is because nature delivers a variety of information to our cells that work in combination to keep us well. And we can't over-estimate the influence of fiber on our colon!

Phytochemicals are so numerous that science cannot isolate all of them…or even name specifically what they all do. But what science does know is that when you put them all together, they make us healthier. Begin to call them your "friendly rainbow" to good health and better numbers – you know your phytonutrient friends by their colors. Fruits, vegetables, legumes (beans and peas), and grains are brilliant with color that is the direct expression of the kinds and amounts of phytochemicals they contain. If it's fresh produce, and colorful, eat it for excellent health.

Plant colors actually come from the process of the plants protecting themselves. Plants make anti-oxidants to strengthen and protect themselves, and this process produces hundreds of these healthy compounds, known as phytochemicals, that feed our cells. Some compounds that have been identified as more notable for their benefits include: Flavonoids, such as saponins and quercitin; Ellagic acid; vitamin E and C; and Beta-Carotene.

This is why a diet that contains an abundance of fruits, veggies and whole grains is promoted by physicians and nutritionists. Inviting as many plants to your plate as you can will enhance your outcomes. In nearly 20 years of working with people to promote healthy lifestyle choices, I have seen the good results in the participants' bodies and their numbers. They've happily reported better numbers when getting blood work updated to check cholesterol and other clinical guidelines. And they feel and look better, too.

Please note that while some of these phytonutrients are available in supplements, the health benefits are better delivered through whole-food consumption. The following list is just some of the highlights of the many benefits of plants:

- Apples: Flavonoids – protect against cancer, lower cholesterol.
- Beans: Flavonoids (saponins) – protect against cancer, lower cholesterol.
- Berries: Ellagic acid – Prevent abnormal cellular changes that can lead to cancer.
- Broccoli: Indoles, isothiocyanates – protect against cancer, heart disease and stroke.
- Carrots and Sweet Potatoes: Beta-carotene – works as an antioxidant.
- Citrus fruits: Falvonoids (limonene) – Antioxidant, inhibit tumor formation, decrease inflammation.
- Flaxseed: Isoflavones – protect against cancer, lower cholesterol.
- Garlic and Onions: Allium (allyl sulfides) – protect against certain cancers and heart disease, boost the immune system.
- Grains: Isoflavones – proctect against cancer, lower cholesterol.
- Red Grapes (and wine) and Tea: Flavonoids (quercitin) – protect against cancer and heart disease.
- Soy (soy beans): Isoflavones – protect against cancer and heart disease, strengthen bones.
- Tomatoes: Flavonoids – protect against cancer, fight infection.

From Mouth to Colon
Avoid the Bloat

Do you have bloating, abdominal discomfort, uncomfortable fullness, heartburn, or nausea? You may be suffering from chronic indigestion or constipation. These health issues can be caused by overeating, eating too quickly and consuming certain foods and beverages triggers this condition.

Emotional factors, such as anxiety or stress, and digestive illnesses, such as pancreatitis, may also contribute to digestive discomfort. A healthy diet, limited in foods that worsen your symptoms, or the addition to foods that strengthen you digestion system can help prevent or alleviate these health concerns. For best results, you may need to seek specified guidance from your doctor or dietitian before altering your diet.

It is important to understand that the quality of your assimilation (how you up-take foods you eat into your digestive system) and elimination (how well the body moves the toxins from your system) plays a big role in determining the quality of your health.

There is a bigger picture in digestive health. Avoiding constipation is key because toxins build up in your system. Eliminating toxins are essential in maintaining healthy digestion. Focus on fresh foods. As a society we can tend to be weak in eating fruits and vegetables.

Good bacteria called probiotics are stimulated in the digestive track by including fresh fruits and vegetables. Yogurt also adds good bacteria….meat and potatoes do not.

Supplement containing acidophilus and bifidobactia are available in drug stores and health food stores, and are especially helpful for gas, bloating, flatulence, diarrhea, and irritable bowel syndrome.

So what can you do to make sure that you are improving your digestion? It turns out that we must pay attention to both ends of the digestive tract…namely mouth and colon.

Do you tend to "inhale" your food? Begin by starting to take smaller bites and thoroughly chew food. You may even want to repeat silently to yourself while you are chewing, "chew, chew, chew," in the beginning to remind yourself to slow down while eating. It is important to get digestive enzymes from your saliva to saturate what you are chewing.

Also, mindful eating is a training process developing awareness of eating patterns. You can put your fork down in between bites or even try using chop sticks which really breaks the habit of wolfing down your meals.

Dietary fiber is also a must to avoid constipation. Remember there is an advantage to including water-soluble beans to your diet. Also include dried fruit such as prunes, figs and dates, and the proverbial daily apple.

Ground flax seed meal is also great because it can keep you "regular" and also provides good Omega-3 fatty acids.

It is important to note that 25 to 50 percent of digestive ailments can be modified, or even prevented by proper eating. If you are not currently including the following in your diet, beginning to slowly introduce items from this list can make a difference in the quality of how you digest your foods and stimulate regular elimination.

Bring the following foods into your daily/weekly menu: yogurt, brown rice, tofu, dandelion greens, sunflower seeds, sea vegetables, flax seed or flax seed oil, papaya, bananas, garlic, turmeric (anti-septic), basil (anti-infection), and sage (anti-inflammatory). Also, it is important to avoid coffee, tea, sodas, and other caffeinated or carbonated drinks. Alcohol, tobacco, chocolate, peppermint, pickled foods, tomatoes, tomato-related products, and all fried or fatty foods can be linked to indigestion. Additionally, citrus fruits and juices are known to cause indigestion due to their acidity.

Hala – What?

I remember, when I was about 12 years old, my grandmother talked about how mint was excellent to chew on because it prevented halitosis. She actually used this word, which expanded my vocabulary, but also horrified me. Some of you may recall what it feels like when you're 12. Talking about bad breath is not a cool conversation. So imagine how I cringed when she was bringing up something as stinky as halitosis.

First of all, what kind of crazy word is that? Wikipedia recounts an interesting legend that suggests that "halitosis" was a made up word by the makers of Listerine to promote their mouthwash in the 1920s. But Wikipedia also confirmed that halitosis is in fact a word with an earlier history, dating back to 1550 B.C., and the mention of bad breath. In those days, it was suggested that a mouthwash of wine and herbs would solve the problem.

So bad breath is not a new affliction. Does anybody have a clothespin? Believe it or not, bad breath follows only periodontal disease and tooth decay, as the third most frequent reason for seeking a dentist. Peee-eeeew!

Gingivitis, abscess, dental cavities, and infection account for the gum and tooth diseases that can contribute to a stinky exhale. Also, infections in the sinuses, nose, throat, tonsils or esophagus can be a smelly culprit. Lung infections and diseases may also play a role in bad breath.

Even if you by-pass the mouth, nose, throat, and lungs, the real problem may be located lower, in the gastrointestinal tract. In this case, bad breath can be disease-oriented, such as GERD (gastroesophageal reflux disease) or intestinal bacterial overgrowth.

Also, extreme cases of dieting will cause imbalances that lead to bad breath. So stay off the starvation diets.

A dry mouth can contribute to bad breath. Regular alcohol use or abuse, tea and coffee, and other drinks that contain caffeine are very drying to the whole body, including the mouth. Certain prescription medications can also make your mouth dry. To combat dry mouth, and that daunting halitosis, do your best to stay hydrated. The recommendation is a minimum of 2 liters of water per day, or eight 8-ounce glasses of water per day.

One of the worse kinds of bad breath, experienced by many people, is "morning breath." This is because our systems shut down while we are sleeping, also causing dry mouth when you wake in the morning. Remember to fight bad breath, stay hydrated.

Herbal teas (my grandmother might suggest fresh mint tea), or other beverages without caffeine, can be included in your daily water in-take. I like to have fresh lemon or lime in my fridge to flavor the water, if your tongue calls for some flavor make it fresh, caffeine-free, and with the least amount of sweetener as possible.

Don't forget the garlic and onions that haunt us hours after they've been eaten. This may be a place for a wise application of chewing gum. I prefer breath mints. Other helpful hints include gargling right before bedtime with mouthwash, tongue cleaning, brushing teeth, flossing and visits to the dentist.

Just a Loaf of Bread Please

Erma Bombeck once said, "The odds of going to the store for a loaf of bread and coming out with only a loaf of bread are three billion to one."

As we all can attest, there is truth about how easy to it is run into the grocery store for one item, and come out with 10. I have become an expert juggler at the grocery store as a result of the extras I grab on the way to the register to buy the one item I stopped to buy. This habit became so chronic that I decided to just grab a cart, no matter what, even if I just wanted to get one item. I figured if I ended up at the register with only a loaf of bread in my cart, no one would mind.

However, I must say sometimes I get a few strange looks when I attempt to stack several things on top of each other using my chin to hold them all in place working my way towards the check out…and yes there is always a line when I am in this delicate juggling act. Have you been there too?

This brings me to another popular topic regarding what we buy at the grocery store. How you can buy healthy and still stay within budget. There is a perception that buying healthy food is more expensive. This can be true for organic produce, but overall, swapping certain processed and packaged foods for others that are healthier add up to about the same cost.

Start with focusing more on whole grains and legumes. Both are nutrient dense and can be substituted for the more empty-calorie snacks that you have available for friends and family. If you are willing to buy the specials in the produce aisle, and you stay out of the snack aisle, you are adding phytonutrients to your cart found in grapes, apples, pears. Look for the sale.

Then head to the cracker section. I like whole wheat Melba Rounds, or pick up whole grain crackers instead of the bag of corn chips…or if you love corn chips, look for the baked variety and eat them with jarred black bean salsa (a vegetable protein). Include these with a chunky garden salad for dinner. You will be cutting meat out of your diet that night, which is inflammatory to the body, and to your grocery bill.

Meat is a major expense to put on the table. You can cut back on meat consumption by using beans for your protein, canned are under $2.00 per can, and dried are even cheaper.

Eggs are also excellent to eat for lunch or dinner and they are inexpensive for the nutritional value they deliver. Eggbeaters are also good if you are watching your cholesterol. You get your protein. You can sauté whatever veggies you like 5 to 7 minutes before you add the scrambled eggs, egg whites or egg substitute. Then top with a little fat free cheese. It makes a delicious and inexpensive meal.

It is very important to buy foods with more than one meal in mind. Fat-free cheese slices can be used in your eggs, for a snack with your whole grain crackers, or melted on your whole grain toast for breakfast or a snack. The same is true when buying produce. Choose varieties with more than one meal in mind so that you are getting the most from your healthy purchases.

King, Prince and Pauper

I've recently discovered that people who live to be 100 years old tend to be breakfast eaters. Stats also show that breakfast eaters are less likely to be smokers or excessive drinkers.

Breakfast literally means "breaking the fast" after you've been dormant for 7or 8 hours. Breakfast supplies almost 25 percent of daily energy expenditure. You need fuel to get your day going with vim and vigor. No one likes dragging through the day....but you might be feeling that way, if you're skipping breakfast.

Studies suggest that 65 percent of your calorie intake should be consumed before 3 p.m. There is a saying, "Eat like a king for breakfast, like a prince for lunch and like a pauper for dinner. "

If you are a breakfast eater, look at what you are eating for breakfast. I used to be a cheerios and strawberries eater in the morning. When my triglycerides went up, I found out that the cereal with berries are considered "double carbs"...a no-no for beginning the day. I wasn't getting any protein in that combo. So, now I eat an egg white omelet, hard boiled egg or whole wheat waffle with peanut butter.

When looking at your health goals, look at your breakfast. If you are still tuned into the all American breakfast with buttered toast, hash browns and breakfast meats you may be starting out with a full belly but you may not be doing your body good in the long run.

Consider rethinking breakfast. I know many people who have made the switch to healthier alternatives and they feel the great results.

You should try to get 30 grams of protein for breakfast. If you cut out breakfast meats to reduce inflammation-causing saturated fat, go for Greek yogurt, reduced-fat cottage cheese, or try switching over to turkey bacon or turkey sausage. The alternative breakfast meats can be higher in added sodium, but will reduce calories from fat.

Breakfast eaters also have a better immune system. Eating breakfast has been linked to boosting anti-oxidants called "gamma interferon," which is a natural anti-viral that will activate your immune system. Alternatively, skipping breakfast has been shown to drop your immune defenses.

So, why all of the talk about breakfast? There are so many health benefits, especially if you choose wisely. Changing up your breakfast can be the thing to focus on to balance your hormones and achieve a healthy weight.

Commit to starting your day with the wisdom of breakfast. This is a worthy habit to start, and you'll reap the rewards. Perhaps you'll have to get up 20 minutes earlier, if you currently aren't getting breakfast in. Maybe you will be inspired to grocery shop differently.

Many healthy breakfast foods can sub for snacks or meals throughout the day. The healthy choices for breakfast such as egg beaters, eat oatmeal with pecans, buckwheat-walnut pancakes or "breakfast" smoothies, can also be tally healthy points throughout the day. Make sure you still intake enough fiber and good carbs with your protein throughout the whole of your day. Peanut butter on apples, or a peanut butter and banana sandwich is also an option.

Breaking the fast with wise choices is the easiest way to ensure that you get all of the health benefits that ward off disease. Positively starting the day with good fuel is like an affirmation for the body. You are instilling the message that you acknowledge the support you get to live and breathe and create in the world with what you choose to focus on first. Your body's health is the gold that helps you achieve your life-long dreams.

Smile For Your Health

If you need to cheer up, just remember, a smile is a curve that sets everything straight. According to experts, smiling is our first facial expression as a baby. Smiling is often contagious and can have a medicinal effect on you and those around you.

Studies have shown that smiling releases endorphins, natural painkillers, and serotonin. Together these three biological chemicals make us feel good. Smiling is a natural drug. Research has shown that forcing yourself to smile when you're sad will actually elevate your mood. In eastern cultures, the practice of the "inner smile" is used to charge the organs and send this positivity to body systems to maintain health and balance. Can you imagine smiling to your liver?

It may sound far-fetched but sending a smile to your liver regularly can boost liver function. Emotions affect the organs. Stress, anger and frustration affect the digestive system and liver function. Among its most important jobs, the liver cooperates with your digestive system to help properly digest all fats, proteins, and carbohydrates. It also works steadily to thoroughly detox your body and keep your body in balance by cleansing and detoxifying almost two quarts of blood *every minute*. That's dedication. So sending a little smile to the liver is a form of appreciation.

This busy organ and has many functions. The liver helps create amino acids which are the building blocks of proteins, and regulates blood glucose levels, and synthesizes cholesterol and triglycerides (fats). Also, the liver creates bile, which is necessary for the proper absorption of fats and essential vitamins, breaks down hormones, toxic substances, and medicines so they can be safely removed from the body, and synthesizes the hormone required to regulate blood pressure.

Stressful living compromises the liver. Poor dietary habits such as including too much sugar, food additives, caffeine, and alcohol will also over-burden this already hard-working organ. Support your liver with getting enough vitamin A and D. Egg yolks and salmon are great sources. Also eat liver supporting vegetables such as garlic, onions, kale, cabbage, cauliflower, broccoli, and Brussels sprouts. Think of supporting your liver when you eat grapefruit, apples, bananas, grapes, pears, pineapple, watermelon and avocado. Cinnamon, turmeric and milk thistle are excellent for the liver, also.

So let's go back to smiling to support your hard-working liver. "When people activate muscle groups that link to specific emotions, their body will react as though they are really experiencing that emotion. If you wrinkle your nose and narrow your eyes your body will release some adrenaline and your heart rate may speed up as though you are angry. If you mimic a smile by lifting the creases of your lips and squinting your eyes, your body will release serotonin, dopamine, and other 'feel-good' indicators," according to positivepsychologynews.com.

The traditional inner smile meditation is a practice of sitting quietly while smiling inwardly at each of the main body organs to ease emotional and physical tensions. Beginning with just a few minutes per day is another way to bring the practice of meditation into your busy life to help recover and bring balance to your mind and body.

Sitting in a chair, place your right hand on the right side of your abdomen, just below your rib cage. Close your eyes and begin to breathe, slowing and lengthening the inhalations and exhalations. Bring a relaxed smile to your face. Focus your internal intention on feeling good and allow your inner smile to radiate from within you to your liver. The idea here is that you take time while meditating to smile inwardly, sending the good feelings to activate a sense of loving-kindness. This will ease both emotional and physical tensions, which will send a thank you to your liver, or wherever you need to support imbalance, pain or injury.

I'm Possible

The classic, one of a kind, Audrey Hepburn said, "Nothing is impossible, the word itself says – I'm possible." Now, that's a positve perspective. I've been a life-long fan of Audrey Hepburn, as much as I'v been a life-long fan of positivity.

A positive frame of mind is a treasure trove that goes deeper than just thinking positive or happy thoughts. The limitless nature of positive thinking creates an abundant foundation for infinite resources and outcomes. I don't know about you, but when I'm feeling my worst I feel limited, stuck and without options. It feels like I'm stuck in a box. Positive thinking lends to an open perspective which is personally practical because it becomes the doorway or window out of the box. A negative point of view keeps the lock on the door, even if one can be found.

If I don't yet know my answer to challenging circumstance, I'm sure I'm going to find the solution. This is personal resiliency is planted deep in self-esteem, self-trust and an attitude grown out of the knowledge that life is inherently good.

Livestrong.com points out, "Misconceptions about positive thinking abound, probably because of its misleading name. A more accurate name for the type of positive thinking espoused by psychologists may be 'constructive thinking.' Positive thinkers reject groundless optimism in favor of brutal realism, yet approach unpleasant realities with a problem-solving attitude rather than a 'don't look for a match and simply curse the darkness' mentality."

Simply stated, the bad fruit of negative thinking tends to be more darkness and negativity. Could it be that some people like the taste, smell and feelings of bad fruit? Productive positive thinking isn't reaching for the keepsake of hopefulness, but aimed at developing real solutions to challenges that can improve or enhance the quality of life, and resolve resistance or conflict.

Statistically, the average person generates 25,000 to 50,000 thoughts per day. That's a lot of thinking. If you are a negative thought processer, I encourage you to train your mind for constructive thinking. In truth, each of us has the opportunity to take control of our outlook on life. This develops a skillful use of mind which fuels many health benefits.

Mayo clinic Researchers continue to explore the effects of positive thinking and optimism on health. Health benefits that positive thinking may provide include:

- Increased life span
- Lower rates of depression
- Lower levels of distress
- Greater resistance to the common cold
- Better psychological and physical well-being
- Reduced risk of death from cardiovascular disease

Constructive positive thinking enables stronger coping skills which fuels empowerment in stressful situations. This stress hardy dynamic reduces the harmful health effects of stress on the physical and emotional bodies. Studies show that positive and optimistic people also tend to live healthier lifestyles — they get more physical activity, follow a healthier diet, and don't smoke or drink alcohol in excess.

"We know why optimists do better than pessimists. Optimists are not simply being Pollyannas; they're problem solvers who try to improve the situation," said psychologist Michael F. Scheier, reflecting on his groundbreaking 1985 research. He provided the scientific framework for exploring the real power of optimism that continues today.

"Think whatever makes you truly happy to think," advises Gerald Jampolsky, author of, *Teach Only Love*. With awareness you can reconstruct your constructive thinking. You can recognize and identify negative thinking patterns, and replace them with encouraging, realistic and productive thoughts which, in turn, will activate healthier living.

Beyond Survival

Understanding why you eat, beyond survival, is very important to making changes that can impact your health. Some of the varieties of reasons we eat include, availability, personal preference, tradition, temptation, social pressure, emotions, and convenience.

If you consider each of these as you monitor your current habits, you may find that you touch on several or all of these reasons for your eating style.

When it comes to availability and convenience there can be a tendency to reach for packaged foods that are quick and easy…or anything else because it is right there at our fingertips. Whatever is quick and on hand becomes what feeds our bodies.

The way to improve this pattern is to make sure ahead of time that you have healthy food in your refrigerator or cupboards so that the food that you have available meets your goals. This is a more healthful approach to fueling your body and mind. Make a shopping list of food essentials and always have them available in your kitchen.

Personal Preference plays a huge role in what you eat…taste, texture and what comforts you has to be looked at here. You can modify your food choices to meet your preferences. Try veggie cheese slices (soy cheese) if you are a regular cheese eater. This does not melt as well, so a grilled cheese sandwich would be out, but if you are willing to eat a PepperJack or Cheddar soy cheese sandwich with lettuce and tomato, you will be switching animal fat for plant-based fat, which heals inflammation, and you won't be grilling the sandwich in butter. Just add a little mustard or fat-free mayo and enjoy!

Tradition is another stumbling block on the road to making a difference in your eating patterns. If you've always eaten a certain food to celebrate holidays, can you change it up to meet your goals? With my Polish background, we eat perogies on Christmas Eve. We hold the butter to a bare minimum, and I now serve non-fat sour cream or fat-free plain Greek yogurt with them. Delicious…no one complains.

Temptation…it speaks for itself. If you are easily tempted away from your eating goals, it is wise to carry an item with you that will satisfy you when you want to cheat. I know a woman who takes a defatted peanut butter (Better 'N Peanut Butter) and jelly sandwich in her purse. She loves this simple sandwich and it is with her at all times. She doesn't have to eat the brownie…or whatever else is showing up to steer her off course.

It can be a real challenge if you go out to lunch or to an event, such as a wedding, with friends or family if they are eating foods that you know will not meet your goals. They may try to sway you to join in, yes this is social pressure. The best trick to stay true to your goals is to eat ahead of time. Therefore, you are there for the socializing ONLY, and can leave the debate of what you are eating out of the conversation. No pressure.

If you understand that eating and emotions go together for you, it is very important to make sure the foods you have available feed your body so you do not overload on empty or high fat calories. You may also want to learn more about stress management, which will help you to manage your emotions differently.

Convenience is also a major downfall to anyone focusing on healthy habits. Fast food can "amp up" your calories because of the high fat and sodium content. It is advised that you look at your time management if this is one of your unhealthy habits. If you are always grabbing fast foods, it may be time to look at how to arrange time in your schedule to eat whole foods...mindfully managing to eat more fresh, nutrient dense foods takes a little more time.

Quiet Your Tummy Woes

Regular quiet time is needed if you are suffering from stomach issues. Acid reflux can be triggered by a number of factors, including certain medications, foods or even stress. If you've ever suffered with a bout of acid reflux, it can be more than just uncomfortable.

According to the American Gastroenterological Association, "one in 10 Americans experiences heartburn or some type of acid reflux symptoms at least once per week." That is a significant number of the population that is affected by digestive issues, some of which may be the result of unhealthy lifestyle habits. If you have irregular eating habits or irregular bathroom habits, or if you experience a lot of stress (real or perceived), you may be contributing to your indigestion.

Before we consider lifestyle habits, we'll look at three types of health conditions that can cause "heartburn" symptoms. Depending on your severity and type, you may want to consider more than lifestyle and over-the-counter solutions. You may want to consult your doctor.

First, "Acid Indigestion" causes a burning sensation in the chest or throat and is due to a reflux of acid in the stomach. It is often referred to as heartburn. It is a condition we all may relate to when we occasionally have discomfort from eating something that doesn't agree with our stomach. It is short-term occasional discomfort is also known as indigestion.

Gastro Esophageal Reflux Disease, or GERD, is a more chronic condition. If you have coughing or difficulty swallowing that is accompanying heartburn symptoms you may want a physician follow up, since GERD can lead to narrowing of the esophagus or ulcers. Stomach acid may be eroding soft tissues, leading to disease.

GERD is a condition where acids in the stomach flow backwards into the esophagus because a valve called the esophageal sphincter (located between the stomach and the esophagus) does not close properly. The stomach acid does not stay in the stomach and flows back up into the esophagus. Symptoms associated with this kind of acid reflux include vomiting or a sour taste in the back of the mouth.

Lifestyle considerations that may contribute to the cause of your heartburn symptoms, include the amount of stress in your life, what you are eating, the way you are eating, or sedentary lifestyle habits which may be adding to your health condition. You might think that spicy foods are common contributors to acid reflux. However, coffee or teas, alcohol, fried or fatty foods, chocolate and citrus juices are the more common culprits that cause discomfort in dietary choices. Look at your consumption of these foods.

Experts say cottage cheese, a baked sweet potato or broiled chicken are all better choices to reduce acid reflux, if you are experiencing an episode. Try to include probiotics in your diet, such as eating yogurt, or talk to your doctor about taking acidophilus supplements, which can be purchased at drug stores or local health food stores to help balance your digestive system. Drinking peppermint tea or using peppermint oil can also be helpful in alleviating stomach upset. Increase fiber consumption for constipation.

Simple habit changes such as eating smaller portions can improve your symptoms. Too much food at one time is a major contributor, so admit your habits if you tend to over-eat. Tight clothing will also play a role in digestive discomfort. Loosen your belt and/or wear looser pants. Make an effort to get regular exercise. Daily movement can help balance digestion. Just 15 to 30 minutes per day of walking can be the healthful habit to get digestion on track.

Also consider if you are getting enough "you" time. It is very important to make enough time for yourself. Slow down, calm your systems. If you are having digestive issues it is essential to set aside regular time, preferably every day, to slow down and relax.

Organic quiet time and space is so needed if you are suffering from stomach ailments. Unplug by quietly sitting alone (away from the television or other electronic devices). Now, focus your attention on becoming calm and grounded by breathing slower, rhythmic breaths through your nostrils. Five minutes daily to start. This simple, yet powerful habit can quickly become the dose of "medicine" your nervous, respiratory, circulatory and digestive systems all need to return to harmony and balance.

The Bend in the Road

It's not the mountain that we conquer but ourselves. This is true in the challenge that is facing us as individuals and as a nation when it comes to our health.

The Academy of Nutrition and Dietetics has a named "the total diet approach," as the foundation of a healthy lifestyle. This dietetic organization is indicating that dietitians recognize that diet education alone is not enough to assist in national efforts to address obesity in the United States. In the guidelines for healthy living, the total diet approach is the combination of physical activity and consuming a balanced variety of nutrient-rich foods and beverages in moderation are at the core of educating the American population.

During March, in recognition of National Nutrition Month, continued education to bring attention to Dietary Guidelines for Americans indicates staggering statistics showing both the resistance to change and challenge of compliance are crippling our

American Culture. Research about American habits posted in 2013 showed:

- 82 percent don't want to give up foods they like in order to eat healthier
- 68 percent don't eat fruits or vegetables at least twice per day
- 62 percent have no time to track their diet
- 60 percent juggle both work and family; prefer to prep meals in less than 15 minutes
- 36 percent have no leisure time for physical activity

This means that most Americans don't meet the guidelines that have been suggested by the Academy of Nutrition and Dietetics. What influences eating practices? Tastes and preferences are a number one excuse for resistance to change and non-compliance. In other words the prevalent attitude is, "I like what I like, and I don't like what I don't like." This may seem a little short-sighted but the stats suggest this stubborn streak is a leading hindrance plaguing the "American way."

Your limitations are whatever excuses block you from actively making choices to protect and maintain your valuable health. These limitations may become your liabilities. Other factors that influence eating practices include, taste and food preferences, body image, time and convenience, environment including home, school and work, and culture including heritage and religion.

"It boils down to making wise food choices in the context of the total diet...focus on variety, moderation and portion sizes," advises the Academy of Modern Dietetics.

How do you get beyond your limitations that are putting you in those large percentages of American unwilling or unable to maintain healthy ranges in diet and exercise? You can begin to see the experts' recommendations as fuel to move you from your constraints and make new choices, which will become the vehicle on your road to freedom. You can create opportunity for freedom from pain, freedom from obesity, and freedom from threat of disease or risk of disease. Freedom in the form of better health lends to feeling and moving better through life.

As Ralph Waldo Emerson said, "We acquire the strength we have overcome." A regular review of guidelines along with a review of your habits builds strength into your lifestyle. Falling into unhealthy patterns does not have to become a problem when you review your own combinations of snags and shortcomings. They are often personal.

We are better able to begin following wise advice for improving our health and quality of life after seriously looking at habits. Success in changing habits is more likely with an attitude of willingness. Start by being willing to stop and take look. Then, listening and applying a personalized variation of the guidelines that will still meet most of your preferences can deliver promising results in your health.

It is said that a bend in the road is not the end of the road…unless you fail to make the turn. We all have the gift in this country of freedom of choice. Can we as the greatest nation in the world take the bend in the road that is asking each of us to make choices to take care of our most precious personal resources…our health?

S-U-P-E-R Food

Nutrition experts are now pointing to a little seed, that has been better known since the 1980's, as a quirky houseplant, naming it the "newest" super food.

Remember the Chia Pet? Still available today, the variety of popular clay figures grows the illusion of hair as the plants sprout when the chia seed paste is watered. FYI… About 500,000 Chia Pets are sold every year in the U.S. as novelties or houseplants!

Now there's evidence that health can spring from these tiny little seeds as well. The chia seed is capable of igniting a powerful boost towards good health. A relative of mint, Native American cultures in the U.S., and many parts of Mexico, have grown and used this plant, for centuries.

A one-ounce serving of chia seeds contains 9 grams of plant-based fat, 5 milligrams of sodium, 11 grams of dietary fiber and 4 grams of protein, according to the USDA. The seeds also have 18% of the recommended daily intake of calcium, 27% phospherous and 30% maganese. Pow! The benefits continue. Chia seeds contain a complete plant-based protein, fiber, omega 3 fatty acids, anti-oxidants, and minerals (magnesium and potassium).

The recommendation is to eat 1 to 2 teaspoons daily, adding them to any food or liquid. It's that simple. Note that the Omega-3 oils in chia seeds, by weight, deliver more healing benefits than salmon. That is a stat worth noting. The inclusion of these essential fatty acids to your diet will also help you to lose weight. Studies showed that those who included omega-3 (from any source) lost 2 pounds more monthly than those who did not.

The chia seed helps mindful eaters to succeed because it expands when mixed into liquid, creating a gel around each seed. This acts as a thickener creating a full feeling and curbing hunger for hours. Cravings are curbed due to this plumping affect, while increasing the amount of vitamins and minerals. This fills not only the tummy but vitamin and mineral recommendations as well.

Chia may be an excellent addition to your daily diet if you have diabetes, or need to regulate your blood sugar levels. Due to the gelling action when met with moisture, both the soluble and non-soluble fiber of the seeds help to slow the conversion of starches to sugar. This creates a constant delivery of energy to get you through your day without feeling lulls or a dip in blood sugar.

Anyone with diverticulitis, diverticulosis, or bowel irregularity will gain from the high fiber content of chia seeds. The outside of the seed is protected by the insoluble fiber, which is unable to be digested and helps food to move smoothly through the digestive process. The gel coating from hydrated seeds keeps the colon moist to also move food along the digestive track.

Wait, there's still more. The chia's ability to deliver high amounts of anti-oxidants gives them trumping power over other similar, seeds such as sesame or flax. While other seeds tend to become rancid easily, chia seeds can be stored at room temperature, ready to eat for up to two full years due to the high amount of antioxidants they contain. Amazing!

You don't have to over-do it. We don't want to flirt with colon disaster. Remember just 1 to 2 teaspoons per day will give you all of these benefits. That's what I call "S-U-P-E-R."

Learn to Float on Trust

How can you keep you own sinking heart afloat during challenging times? My life preserver is faith, knowing and trusting in God, even when I don't understand the plan. Faith is how I get through the "not knowing," and I like to pair it with trust to help me to develop a stronger sense that, even without all of the answers, the answers are on their way. There is safety in this positive expectancy.

With faith you can feel confident to maintain your composure, explore and consider new options, if need be, and be ready for the blessing you are getting prepared to receive. If you are in the not-knowing of a situation it's easy, even natural, to feel anxiety, worry, concern, angst…if any of these sound familiar, it's time to develop faith and trust.

Sometimes life can get bleak. Feeling like life has no direction is quite normal during periods of change. An "aimlessness" can emerge. The hidden treasure of aimlessness is the opportunity to get into life's boat and go with the flow choosing positivity to see where you end up. But aimless meandering without hope can lead to depression. If you get stuck make sure you share your concerns. It's not healthy to keep worries inside.

Remember that meandering through life a while requires letting go, which can be hard when the bills need to be paid, you feel responsible to relationships, or you just lack a fondness for change. Admit when you are clutching on and white knuckling it. Sometimes you've got to fake it 'til you make it. Which brings us back to trust.

One way that you build trust, if you feel it is in short supply, is to create a positive present moment affirmation. Affirming what is true and good, and what you expect from life will stomp on those feelings that are feeding you negativity through anxiety and worry, and establish feelings of confidence, positive expectancy and self-assurance.

In the beginning, it is important to tune into how you are feeling without resisting the fear of the unknown. Facing the unknown is scary. The purpose of positive affirmations is to evoke new, more manageable feelings that will help you go with the flow of life instead of resisting it. State positively what you would like to be true for you.

The first time you say, "I am living in full faith and trust," you may feel doubtful, numb, cynical, unworthy, skeptical or a myriad of other feelings that do not resonate with living, faith or trust. You have just uncovered all of the parts of you that don't resonate with this self-empowering statement. That's good. Physical sensations you might feel with these attitudes can include, nausea, queasiness, tension, or hyperventilation, and your fear may over ride your positive statement with something that feels like, "I am doomed."

This is all perfectly normal when you are meeting your fear. That is the added benefit of creating any powerful positive affirmation. It measures how well you are aligned to the feeling behind the positive energy you are conditioning yourself to live by.

You get a reflection of how much your statement is alive and active inside by how much you feel it to be true. When you can say, "I am living in full faith and trust" and you feel calm, peace, good will, joy and gratitude, even without knowing what might happen next, you know you are aligned completely with this statement as your truth.

You may need to practice saying your affirmation several times per day, internally (silently) and aloud, until you do feel it as your personal statement of truth in your body and mind and emotions. When you own any positive affirmation, it becomes totally true for you. You'll begin to notice that life meets and greets you differently, and you'll find new direction, deepen life's meaning, and expect a promising future.

The Sugar Monkey

I know a woman who has a wonderful way of describing her challenge of controlling her sugar cravings. She often says, "I have the Sugar Monkey on my back."

Do you have the Sugar Monkey on your back? Do you crave sugar? Do you love to indulge in decadent sweets? Do you dream about that next delicious sweet confection blasting your taste buds?

The good thing about the idea of the "Sugar Monkey" is that it gives you the opportunity to imagine your sugar craving outside of your need for sugar. It has a new name, "the Sugar Monkey."

If every time you crave a sweet you recognize it as the "Sugar Monkey" riding your back, it gives the reach for a sweet a new perspective, and perhaps the will to say "no." Creating some space between your urge for the sweet, and reaching for the sweet, is only a Sugar Monkey away. Consider creating one.

If you're willing to give imagery a try you will be able to create a new perspective about your sugar craving. In this way, you can become more aware of your obsession with sugar (or any other craving) by approaching it in a new way.

Name your Sugar Monkey, visualize how it looks in detail. Is it cute…or does it have gnashing teeth that demand sugar? You may realize your first step is to tame your Sugar Monkey, if you feel it is vicious or demanding. You may have to include the befriending of your Sugar Monkey in your imagery.

The more detail you give your imagery, the more personal and powerful it will become. Telling the Sugar Monkey "no" may be much more effective than trying to tell yourself "no" when you're having a craving.

If you were able to tell yourself "no" more effectively, you wouldn't feel burdened about your cravings. However, just like teaching a puppy to stay in its own yard, you can teach your Sugar Monkey to reach for a better sweet. Disciplined monkeys tend to eat more fruit…apples, oranges, bananas, pears and occasional sweets. You can train your Sugar Monkey to be your ally instead of the enemy. You are the trainer.

So what causes sugar cravings? Sometimes there are hormonal and chemical imbalances that will trigger cravings. You can check with your doctor to rule these out or get some medical advice.

Secondly, the truth is that sweets tastes good. It can be that simple. If you have an inclination toward the gratification of sweet flavors, especially from a young age, it is more of a challenge for you to eat the wider range of other flavors that you have available to you.

If your tongue is dialed up to high on the sweets scale, you will have to use determination to train those taste buds to receive alternate information. But that is what a Sugar Monkey is for! Go for naturally occurring sweets instead of always eating the high sugary snacks. Your sugar monkey might eventually even like eating more veggies.

According to the American Heart Association Americans consume an overabundance of sugar, averaging about 22 teaspoons of added sugars per day. The recommendation is to limit added sugars to about 6 teaspoons per day for women and 9 for men.

Other ways to train your Sugar Monkey away from cravings include:

- Get up and go. Take your Sugar Monkey for a walk.
- Regular and consistent eating habits will ensure you don't get too hungry.
- Chew gum.
- Becoming friendly with your habits

Taste Bud Confusion

If you are attempting to eat healthier, you may be suffering from taste bud confusion. In our culture, we can be inundated artificial flavors, and added salts and fats that are poured into packaged and fast foods. When you are committed to the experience of the salty crunch…or the sponginess of the cake…or the cookie that melts in your mouth, fresh unprocessed foods can cause full-mouth revolt.

That is part of the problem isn't it? Natural, unaltered foods deliver a different kind of conversation to the tongue. Whole fresh foods whisper instead of scream. We've been conditioned to expect that flavors should blast our palette. Whole foods are more subtle.

If your doctor has suggested to you that you change your diet, or you are considering doing this by your own choice, I urge you to slowly begin to refine your tasting skills. Raw veggies with fat free dip can become the new crunchy. Not the same salty greasy crunch you may be used to if potato chips are a favorite snack, but if you make this a habit you will learn to appreciate the natural goodness that fresh veggies deliver in taste.

Sugar snap peas and raw carrot sticks are pleasant and mellow. Red and yellow peppers are also offer a delicious sweetness that is unique. The coolness of the cucumber and the zesty conversation that a tomato leaves on your tongue requires discernment.

The suggestion of enjoying these flavors may be more in tune with seasonal expectations. In this area of the country (Northeast) farm fresh produce is ample in the summer. This is when we expect the flavors of fresh tomatoes, corn on the cob, cucumbers, and peppers to be at their peak...many people look forward to this.

Fresh produce is usually more expensive in winter months because it is not locally grown. The same with fresh fruits…we eat it abundantly in season. Both of these categories are available in the can or frozen varieties making them more affordable. Often if you are buying frozen peppers or onions they also offer convenience because they are already chopped, sliced or diced. You may also want to begin to experiment with herbs and spices, which bring out the natural flavors of foods.

Beverages can also become a challenge when making dietary changes. Many people tell me that, for them, water has no taste. Sodas and other sugary beverages add calories to your daily menu by blasting you with exaggerated flavor and empty calories. Even "diet drinks" are designed to woo your tongue.

However, think about changing your mindset if your habit is to grab this kind of sugary drink with every meal. It may seem far-fetched, but can you consider making water more of a beverage? Here's how.

If you have a Britta filtered pitcher, you can have cold pure water sitting in your fridge where it is more likely to be chosen as a beverage. Adding a slice of lemon or lime to your glass of water can add natural flavor. Be patient. You will adapt in just a few days to the lighter, fresher flavors.

Highest Good Leadership

Making a priority of conflict resolution, rather than winning or being right, makes a leader in creating a better world. A better world is not necessarily a "global" perspective. Developing harmony and collaboration right where you live – in your home, within your family, throughout your community, is no small intention. Develop the attributes of a person who is willing to step beyond personal perspective and self-absorption. Consider the highest good for everyone in the situation, including yourself.

This is a practical suggestion. With so many challenges we each may face each day, wouldn't it be nice to contribute to a trend of supporting each other and working together. General Douglas MacArthur pointed out, "A true leader has the confidence to stand alone, the courage to make tough decisions, and the compassion to listen to the needs of others. He does not set out to be a leader, but becomes one by the equality of his actions and the integrity of his intent."

Difficult circumstances may be calling you to be a leader. Situations can arise that may allow one person, perhaps you, who is strong in character, willing and able, to steady the ground of disagreement, and utilize the charm of this intention to gracefully establish tone and precedent that will spark resolution and harmony. Personifying this call to follow wisdom takes thinking larger than yourself, and can create positive outcomes that will benefit all involved.

"A disagreement or incident involving someone who's not that important to you, like a guy who cut you off in traffic or a rude cashier, is something that should roll off your shoulders. Save the effort for resolving conflicts with the people you cherish," advises Joel Osteen.

It is good advice to begin to live the intention of leading conflict resolution by letting go of reacting. By releasing emotional responses to situations that do not really matter much to your long-term quality of life, you will actually be developing the attributes of acceptance, patience, easiness and peace of mind, which definitely will contribute much to your real long-germ quality of life and well being.

Acceptance and patience brings more presence to employ the skill of careful listening, contemplating others' needs as well as your own, and naturally bringing the betterment of living well to "the people you cherish" and the culture we all live in.

There is heart in an approach that aspires to find inclusive resolution. Dropping an exclusive outlook, reflecting on a broader view, creates an open mindset that also embraces the feelings behind the interests of others involved. Softening judgment, while considering what others are feeling, takes into account needs and emotions, part of deeper consideration in resolving conflict.

It may seem that only the noble would want to take on this kind of ambassadorship that requires slowing down, and stepping out of your own self interest long enough to listen and feel what meets the good of all involved. Not excluding self-interest, and still evaluating what spark of mediation could deliver a blessing for all, instead of friction…a flash of insight, instead of the clash of disagreement.

Dissolving roadblocks to family, work and community harmony is less about negotiation and mostly about caring for the larger well-being of those you cherish, and that you value. Showing respect in words and actions, and remaining aware of differences are sure tactics for resolving problems faster and with less difficulty.

The Produce Man

How often do you have a great conversation with your produce man? I encourage it. I got quite an explanation about how Organic veggies are handled. I also found out there are certain guidelines about where they can even be located to be sold as "organic."

I was looking for organic kale over the weekend. I already had organic celery, organic baby lettuce, and organic arugula in my cart. I had the good fortune of finding the produce manager in his department.

You could imagine how boring a job might be if you spend more time with veggies than with people. So, he was happy to talk to me. All you produce people out there…get ready. Let the conversations with people begin!

He explained that in order for fruits and veggies to be officially "organic" they have to be handled and displayed separately from others that have been sprayed with pesticides. Therefore, a lot of stores actually have organics (such as the beets that he pointed out to me) but he has no room to separate them so they could not be sold as organic. This is slowly evolving as more people are looking for organic produce.

You may be wondering what all the hype is about when it comes to buying organic fruits and vegetables. If you've seen some of the prices of organics it is likely that you choose your produce based on the common variety and skip organic.

Some research has shown that ingesting too many toxic chemicals from pesticide use can be harmful, and can even lead to disease. Some illnesses evolve over time, such as inflammatory issues or cancer, some are more immediate such as allergic reactions.

So because of what I learned from the produce man, I feel it is safe to purchase and enjoy all of your produce but here are some interesting tips you may want to remember about the "Dirty Dozen" and the "Clean Fifteen."

The Dirty Dozen are the most sprayed with pesticides and it is recommended that you limit them or make every effort to buy organic. These are: Apples, Celery, Strawberries, Peaches, Spinach, Nectarines (imported), Grapes (imported), Sweet Bell Peppers, Potatoes, Blueberries (domestic), Lettuce, Kale/Collard Greens.

The clean fifteen is the list that you do not need to buy organic. They have the lowest amounts of pesticides. These are: Onions, Sweet Corn, Pineapples, Avocado, Sweet Peas, Mangoes, Eggplant, Cantaloupe (domestic), Kiwi, Cabbage, Watermelon, Sweet Potatoes, Grapefruit, Mushrooms.

I always buy what is available but get excited when I can purchase "cleaner" food when I can find it. I don't obsess over my veggies because I just think it is important to get them into my diet. I wish you good health and excellent nourishment.

Think Nothing Of Starting Over
Success Can Be the Value of " Try Again"

I invite you to a 21-Day Challenge (which may take more than 21 days). Whether you are still activating a New Years' resolution, or you have a vision or goal you want to accomplish, you can utilize this template as a powerful meditation tool to start something new.

Affirmation and visualization have been clinically proven to enhance outcomes. So take charge of the power tool of your mind to make a positive difference in your life. The willingness to develop the focus it takes to change is a major part of creating and maintaining new patterns.

The outline of "7 days of quotes" is a template, ultimately to be repeated three weeks in a row, to begin creating the mind power and will to meet your goals. It takes 21 consecutive days of repeating the new pattern to begin to establish a new habit. If you want to create something new you have to focus on it long enough for it to take root and become your new realty. (NOTE: You can also use any quotes that inspire you.)

For most people, realistically it may take more than 21 days to create a new habit or manifest a new dream into your new reality. Old patterns and life circumstances can challenge your resolve. This is why working with the 7 days in a row template can be your structure to change. If you go off-goal at any point, start back at day 1 until you have completed the 7 days of quotes meditations while successfully accomplishing your goal each day.

So the only rule is – Think nothing of starting over – each time acknowledge that you are reinforcing your intention. The reinforcement is adding another layer of strong steel, if you truly are starting over with integrity to establish new patterns.

Day 1 (no matter how many of them you have) is your friend. Day 21 is your destination. Begin again each time you don't accomplish your intention for the next consecutive day until you've mastered your intentions for 21 days in a row. It's a worthy process. Once you've successfully completed 21 days in a row, you will be successfully living your new pattern.

Before you start day one, be clear about the intention, goal or dream you want to accomplish. Launch your intentions with a clear vision of the outcome. Be brave about what you will have to do each day to meet your goal. What will you need to let go of? What actions will you need to take?

Use the power tool of your mind and imagination to see and feel having what you intend. How will you act, think and feel in your new reality?

Don't judge yourself for having to start over. Focus on the meaning behind each of the daily quotes in relation to your vision for success. You will accomplish the 21 days in a row when you are living your goal with ease.

I suggest that you reflect on the quote of the day listed below at two critical points through the day, in the morning before you start your day, and again at the end of the day before you go to sleep. If you want to review through the day as well it will provide extra reinforcement.

Day 1 "When I dare to be powerful – to use my strength in the service of my vision, then it becomes less and less important whether I am afraid."

- Audre Lorde

Day 2 "Concentration is the secret of strength."

- Ralph Waldo Emmerson

Day 3 "The size of your success is measured by the strength of your desire, the size of your dream, and how you handle disappointment along the way."

- Robert Kiyosaki

Day 4 "Failure will never overtake me if my determination to succeed is strong enough."

- Og Mandino

Day 5 "Perhaps I am stronger than I think."

- Thomas Merton

Day 6 "Storms make trees take deeper roots."

- Dolly Parton

Day 7 "Great works are performed not by strength, but by perseverance."

- Samuel Johnson

*REPEAT days 1 through 7, allowing the affirmations to inspire you, until you have met your goals 21 straight days in a row.

Build strength to focus on the actions that bring you what you want. Take time at the beginning of your day to study your daily quote to stay inspired, and reinforce your strategy. Acknowledge at the end of each day, with honesty…how well you are meeting your goals?

What's Your Combo

Ok…I'm going to take combos to a new level. Instead of a "combo meal," let's talk about combinations of activities and movement. Based on your interests and ability to move, how much activity are you getting in a day…and how often during the week?

What's your combo? I am an outside walker, hiking, yoga girl. My dad is a "mall walker," and a walk the dog kind of guy. Some people prefer core-strengthening exercises. Others are into yard work, then, head to the gym to lift weights. There is always the sporty type, committed to conditioning, and then playing their game hard.

I am sure there are numerous households with at least one piece of exercise equipment tucked under the bed, unused. Are you using your treadmill as a clothes rack? If you are, let someone borrow that piece of equipment who may actually use it, and admit that it's not really your calling.

It doesn't have to be all or nothing...instead you can engage in several different activities that you enjoy that can add up to healthy daily movement. Treadmills may not be on your list. Maybe aerobics classes and picking up sticks in the yard is your natural combo. Make the commitment to moving more in your life in ways that are part of your daily living. You can reap the results and lower your chances of being a statistic.

Some people enjoy surfing...the net that is. Unfortunately, this kind of "activity" is far too prevalent in our culture. Too much sedentary activity has led to the staggering statistics sweeping our country contributing to both adult and childhood obesity. Research is showing that in 2008 sixty-six percent of the U.S. population was over-weight. That's two-thirds!

Thirty-two percent of children are overweight, and 17 percent, ages 2 to 19, were obese. The good news is that this health issue, which has been growing exponentially in our culture, began to level off in 2010. Obesity is now holding steady as a health concern at 34 percent. That is still a hefty segment of the population needing to lose weight.

My question for you is -- what is your activity combo? Are you getting the kind of movement in that qualifies you as a "mover" instead of a "sitter"…that is unless you are a baby sitter. It turns out that babysitting is a great way to get more activity.

Young children keep you moving and the good news is, as a service, it can make you money as well as keeping you slim…unless you watch your grandkids. Then, along with the health benefits, while you may not get financial rewards, the benefits of relationship building and the great memories you are creating are their own rewards.

Here are more combos that make up an active lifestyle:

o Babysitting, walking, tennis
o Maintaining the yard, taking the stairs, weights, jumping rope
o Wii fit, swimming, dancing
o Biking, elliptical, Pilates
o Volley ball, Just Dance video dance game
o Walking, stretch bands, jumping jacks
o Running, then core strengthening exercises
o Walking in place in living room during commercials, "curls" with cans of peas
o Hula hooping, jump roping, soft ball

Building your combo taps your health potential. Winning the game of life combines activities and movement that positively defines who you are and can be a statement of the way you live your style. Being "in style" puts you in sync with your health and well-being.

Do You Feel Stuck?

Apathy, a state of non-caring and non-doing, can be a negative force that undermines your ability to successfully meet your intentions and goals. Apathy can contribute to unhappy and unaccomplished living.

To turn this corner, it is important to grasp the understanding that successful people continue moving forward, even when they are met by their own resistance. Resistance is a normal part of creative, productive process. Feel it and keep going.

Awareness is the key to unlock the door to happiness and success. Pay attention to your own behaviors, then, learn to step-by-step move forward without judgment. This tactic can get to the root of what is holding you back and reveal barriers keeping you from achieving your goals.

What are some examples of self-sabotaging behavior? It stems from mindsets or behaviors that undermine your sense of empowerment and feeling you are in control of your success. Forgetting that there is more than one way to accomplish a goal, caring too much about what other people think, not believing that you are worthy enough to meet your goals – all reflect negative thought patterns, which can fuel apathy. With these attitudes, you're likely to remain under motivated and sedentary.

Clarity comes from looking at yourself without judgment, to see where you are stuck. Observe when you are operating out of fear. Bringing awareness to negative patterns is like turning a light on in a dark room.

Start an "awareness list" to bring yourself structure and accountability. It is a sure way to view positive and negative patterns. Write down each activity, thought or emotion that moves you forward. Do the same for the patterns that take you away from your goal.

Yes, this is a time commitment. This takes regular self-review. Get serious by looking deeper and writing down the truth of your feelings, i.e, feeling lost, unlucky, or lazy. Study your excuses such as "I don't know how" or "I don't want to" or "I don't have time." It is good to be accountable to someone that you report into about what you are charting about your patterns. Sharing your observations with a friend or a mentor, or seeking some professional guidance such as a traditional counselor, personal trainer, or personal nutrition counselor once you have a list can bring productive results.

Developing the discipline to pay attention to patterns that undermine your happiness and success is not self-punishment - it is self-empowerment. You'll be glad you cared enough to pay attention and moved into action when you change just one pattern and achieve even one new goal successfully. Your new outcomes can bring you happiness and fulfillment.

Use a Little "Umph"

Have you ever heard the saying, "The only difference between try and triumph is a little 'umph'." Where does "umph" come from? I feel it comes from inside of you. Sometimes when you are tired and overwhelmed by what life is asking, or if you've been working hard to meet a goal still with no end in sight, we can get discouraged.

Turning discouragement into encouragement is a turning point on the road to triumph. If you keep your hopes high you can access the voice of hope in yourself. Sometimes you have to reach deeper, or beyond yourself in order to get a second wind when life feels challenging.

I consider looking for encouragement a kind of "prayer" that you ask from life to keep you going even when you can't see the end yet. Life can give you a positive whisper when you develop an attitude to listen and receive.

Receiving encouragement is rewarding. You don't have to appear needy to accomplish getting moral and emotional support. As a matter of fact, people don't even have to know that you are in the process of raising your own spirits. Encouragement often starts with yourself.

It is healthy to discover what lifts your spirits. It could be whistling a tune, taking a walk, or playing fetch with the dog. What is your secret "umph" ingredient? It is also good to reach out to others to find the encouragement to journey on toward your success. Surround yourself with a good support network.

Triumph is the ultimate in success. Make sure you hunt down negative thoughts, and turn away from negative habits or negative people. These are the secrets of triumph.

"Umph" is another word for talent. Where to you bring that extra umph that leads you to positive contributions and to making a difference? Also, "umph" and passion also go hand-in-hand. Deeply caring about the things that matter to you brings a lot of "umph" to fuel your efforts.

We all know the old adage, "When the going get's tough, the tough get going." There's a lot of "umph" in that attitude. But it is normal to stall out at some point. That's a good time to re-assess and re-group in order to keep up the stamina to meet your goals.

"Hitting the wall" is actually a common setback in any challenge. When you get to the point where you perceive you can't go on any longer you've hit the wall. That's when it's time to freshen-up and re-shape your vision. This helps you to stay current with your goals. You can better do this by reassessing. There is a lot of "ump" in seeking support and feedback from someone you trust.

Remember that your aspirations are worth it. When you re-focus on the value of what you intend, even if it doesn't turn out the way you expect, there is valor in the boldness that you have stepped foot on the path toward your success. Keep the "umph" in trying and triumph will be yours.

Exquisite Living

Exquisite living includes remembering to remember yourself in your busy life. Establish habits in the busy-ness of your week that meet your personal needs and well-being including: healthy eating habits, restorative time, regular exercise, developing and maintaining balanced relationships, living by a great life philosophy, and following your creative flow. The little extra time and effort delivers great results.

For Diet: Include a minimum of one whole grain during at least one meal per day, and eat one serving of whole grain as a snack per day. Eat one of these: baked beans, black beans, kidney beans, chick peas, black eyed peas, pinto beans at least one time per day. Eat one to two pieces of fruit per day. Eat at least one salad per day. Eat at least one cooked vegetable per day. Eat one piece of 70- to 85- percent cocoa chocolate per day (I prefer the Ghiradelli squares...only one!), or other foods high in flavonoids like cranberries, onions, tea or red wine.

For restorative time: Play with your dog, brush your cat, listen to music that relaxes or inspires you, play the piano or other instrument that celebrates your talent (or listen to someone else express their talent to play an instrument or to sing), take a tai chi or yoga class, set aside 15 to 20 minutes a day to stretch and breathe.

Regular exercise: If you are not currently very active, the best approach is to start with 10 minutes and work toward 30 minutes of exercise 6 days per week. You can walk around your dining room table or march in front of the television if it is too cold or snowy to walk outside...just move. Once you reach 30 minutes of aerobics, 6 days, start to include some strength training, such as stretch bands, in your routine.

Developing and maintaining relationships: There is value to feeding good relationships with your time and attention. Verbalize your appreciation to others for what they do. Give a hug or a smile whenever appropriate. Don't be stingy about lending a hand when you can. Say thank you often. Show up with much love and care in your significant other relationships by taking the time to notice how those around you need you most.

Have a great life philosophy: Waking up each day knowing that you intend to make a difference, and intending to receive the gifts that the day will bring, contributes to exquisite living. Some of the oldies but goodies include: "seeing the glass half full", "always do your best," "look on the bright side of life."

Following your creative flow: Make a date with yourself (and only you) at least once per week to do something fun and/or creative. Take one full hour out of your schedule to re-discover what makes you tick. This can give you the depth to manage other demanding situations that come up in life. Find what brings you joy. Do you enjoy looking for unique greeting cards to share? Do you like ice skating, knitting or creating an art or craft? Are you a woodworker? Would you like to learn more about using the computer?

Don't be afraid to make mistakes: To be the best human being you can be, you may not always get it "right," and that's part of being human. Staying connected to the intention to love and make a difference deepens the experience of living. Sometimes being goofy or awkward still delivers an opportunity to communicate, to support, to teach or to learn.

Exquisite living celebrates that you know your worth. The little extra time and effort you take to focus on valuing yourself in all of these areas will deliver more health, more happiness and more joy.

Intend For Positive, Powerful Change

Changing habits is a complete reshaping of your orientation to life as you know it. In order to go in a new direction, and create a different reality, it's important to find your depth. The strength to change comes from the inside. Call your being to new life. You can do it.

It takes more than the will to change. It is more than mind over matter. It is literally a gathering of your life forces. Imagine all of the molecules that you are. That is, imagine a 2 with 27 "zeros" after it. That is the estimate of how many molecules you are.

Now when you make a permanent change in your way of being (break a habit, or command a lifestyle change) all 2×10 to the 27th power of molecules have to shift along with you. So that's like gathering up all of the energy that you are, turning yourself into a "laser for change."

If you are a smoker, you've programmed your 2,000,000,000,000,000,000,000,000,000 molecules to relate to the nicotine. Add your emotions, which can be attached to the smoking experience, and your mind patterns, which can fix you into repeating a convincing need for your hook, and you are a walking talking cigarette.

The same is true if you are addicted to alcohol, or other substances, including the sugary late night snack that you look forward to every night that is contributing to your rising blood sugar and triglycerides.

Please understand that you are wired – programmed – by all of your choices, whether you own them or not. In order for change to truly occur, all of the variables have to be above the radar and coded for change. Facing the below the radar (unconscious) variables, better known as the shadow or "the dark side" is discovering the blueprint to constructing how you operate.

The shadow side of your life can be an underlying sabotaging motivation. For example, if you go to the fridge without really feeling hunger, you may be eating because you are lonely…but you don't register loneliness. You're eating to fill a void. That's the dark side. You shine the light on these patterns by becoming more aware of your actions, and how they undermine your goal.

Successful change comes from deliberately aligning all conditions to be your strength. That includes understanding your choices and actions. Owning your energy leads the way to shape the new model of what you intend to become. For anything you want to change, sometimes you have to let go of the environments and people that another dimension to the conditions that hold you to continue old patterns.

All of your habits, the way you eat, sleep breathe, play, pray, work, move, laugh, grumble, emote, care…are delivering the experience you are having right now. Taking ownership of your whole life force doesn't have to be overwhelming. However, it does ask you to become honest with yourself. Honesty breeds awareness. Awareness uncovers your fear.

Fear is part of this process. Are you afraid you've missed the opportunity to use awareness wisely and sharpen your skills to choose who you can become? You don't have to be led by old, negative patterns. Many professionals including, physicians, registered dieticians, personal trainers, counselors, ministers, massage therapists, physical therapists, and yoga therapists can be on your team of "wise ones" to assist you to shift your attention towards the new you. It's never too late.

And don't forget loving, caring family and friends, that support you. They can also be instrumental as you gather up all of those molecules that you are into one powerful laser beam of intent for positive, powerful change.

You Are Awesome

With so much focus in the media of several installments, over many years, of J.K. Rowling's Harry Potter story, it is safe to guess that even if you haven't seen the movies or read the books, you know who Harry Potter is, and that you can imagine what this young boy must have felt when he was told, "You're a wizard, Harry."

It would be both exciting and a little scary to hear those words. But I am going to say them to you now. You are a wizard. Sometimes you have to get out of your head and into the moment to access your magic.

A friend and I were comparing our weekends. I said I had an awesome weekend. She said she had an awful one. I enjoyed a movie night with friends on Friday. On Saturday, I witnessed the phenomenal triple-crown victory of American Pharaoh while eating a great meal at a Pittsburgh sports bar, and saw a fantastic concert in a small venue, The Carnegie Music Library, with my daughter. Sunday I ran errands, and did some yoga and laundry. (I also managed to pull weeds, trim a tree and work on a creative project over this same weekend.)

My friend on the other hand has a lot on her plate and had to work instead of play all weekend. Yet, we laughed at the fact that we both had "aw" in our weekend. Mine was awesome. Hers was awful. We all have good and bad weekends varying between fun to work. The point is that with reframing your focus away from awful, you too can have an awesome weekend, even if it is all work, work, work.

Yes, you are a wizard. With the magic wand of your own attention, you can still make sure you find time to appreciate life, take a break, make time to laugh, make time to get outside to create some balance. My friend admitted that she took regular intervals to go outside and sit. The weather was nice and she could celebrate the sunshine and awesome summer days. She is quite an awesome wizard, and I am happy to know her.

I saw a poster that said, "Don't judge me. I was born to be awesome, not perfect." There is some real merit in this philosophy that I live by. If you can let go of perfection, you can create awesome moments even in your demanding "awful" circumstances. You don't have to do it "right" to live it well.

Cut yourself a little slack, but not too much. This next perspective may be going a little too far. Have you ever seen a poster that said, "I'm not fat. It's just my awesomeness swelling up inside." Funny.

Yes, it is important to be realistic and to own your challenges. However, the magic wand of a positive perspective offers you the opportunity to liberate your "inner awesomeness" to enhance any situation or challenge. The results will be the unleashing of the "wizardry" of your capacity to create quality living, no matter what the circumstances.

Awesomeness has a name, and that name is YOU. The film critic, Roger Ebert, said, "The Muse visits the act of creation, not before. Don't wait for her. Start alone." It takes you walking those first steps towards the door to get yourself onto the deck to enjoy a small part of an awesome day. Whatever your Muse is, in order to weave awesomeness into your ordinary or demanding moments, it is up to you to remember that you are the keeper of the magic.

I like to live by this kind of wizard thinking -- Never give up on what you really want to do. The person with big dreams is more powerful than one with all the facts – author unknown.

Isn't it true that when you get sucked into the mundane thinking of the ordinary world you can start to feel the weight of a heavy "to do" list. The world can sink to black and white. You tend to polarize toward all or nothing thinking. This is death to a wizard. Bring your colors back to your world with your positivity wand. Take time to smile, breathe, sing, walk or jog…the big dreams are built on those small magical moments of remembering to enjoy your life.

The Right and The Wrong of Sugar

Let me serve you some sugar. Will power is directly related to glucose levels in our brain. Glucose is a simple sugar that is an important energy source and is a component of many carbohydrates. According to the research, the body and brain need glucose. It is the fuel that keeps us going.

So, congratulations. You are not the weak, unfocused freak you thought you were! True will power comes from making sure that your brain is being fed the fuel to keep your mind clear, and your body functioning.

When we deny ourselves food as a weight loss strategy, we actually sabotage our will power! We get stuck in perceiving that we can't activate our own good intentions, when really we are being pushed by the body's drive for fuel.

So toss out the guilt and get eating! The experts are saying that the most important thing we can do when we want to lose weight and get healthy is eat the right carbs to keep our glucose levels consistent.

Your body actually searches for carbohydrates to function. When you ignore or suppress the urge to eat, depriving yourself of fuel, you throw your body into survival mode. Research is finding that the frenzy to eat is not a lack of will power but the body's urgent need to keep glucose levels from plummeting.

This urgency becomes even more intense the longer you go without eating because the body becomes alarmed. You may feel desperate, illogical or aggressive as all of the fight or flight signals drive you to restore your balance the fastest way possible…wolfing down simple carbs. Do you know the feeling?

So the next time you grab those potato chips or fries, or you absolutely must eat your favorite candy bar or piece of cake, it is most likely that you haven't eaten enough. And remember, most fast foods do not deliver the kinds of carbs that are slow release. If you haven't eaten often enough your body may be choosing the fastest solution to keep you functioning. This "hardwire to survive" overrides your goals and intentions.

When your body feels safe, you move beyond the desperate search of carbohydrates to survive, and can resume higher level thought processes such as setting goals, and keeping your intentions.

Complex carbohydrates, also referred to as Low GI (glycemic index) carbohydrates, release slower into your blood stream and can keep your glucose levels stable for 3 hours. Foods such as whole grains, veggies and fruits deliver life-giving carbs to give you plenty of steam to think, be and act in the world without desperately clamoring for a cookie.

The biggest relief is, if you put this nutritional truth into practice, you can still choose a cookie now and then, without fighting with yourself about it. You have found the empowerment of you own balanced glucose levels and you will be more likely to practice excellent decision-making skills.

To begin, you must stop skipping meals, which throws your body into emergency mode. If it means making all of your meals on the weekend so that you are not challenged by time management to have the right foods available, do it!

Meals and snacks matter if you are serious about losing weight and positively influencing your health.

Also, if you start a craving ask yourself, "Was my last meal too long ago? If it is not yet mealtime, choose a wise snack to answer your body's call for fuel. When you properly fuel your body, your body doesn't run you around. You gain the will to meet your goals and feel good about what you are creating for yourself and your health.

Wise Choice Making

Last week I went to Subway for lunch. There was a line but things were moving quickly. The guy next to me ordered a buffalo chicken sandwich. I ordered an egg white sandwich. The sandwich builder asked if I wanted cheese. I said no, thank you.

Buffalo Chicken turned to me in surprise and said, "What! No cheese?"

I said "no thank you." I did not want to spout any facts about what full-fat cheese does to your arteries. It's not my style to lecture in public, unless I'm asked. Also, some people really like cheese.

Buffalo Chicken ordered provolone cheese, lettuce, tomato and extra buffalo sauce on his sandwich. We continued on down the line. I got my usual veggies – lettuce, tomato, onion, cukes, banana peppers (no spinach, it gives me a rash.)

I usually get vinegar, salt and pepper, or the fat-free sweet onion dressing. However, because of Buffalo Chicken, I asked, and discovered that the buffalo sauce was fat free…so I ordered it.

Buffalo Chicken paid his bill, then turned to me and said, "Buffalo Sauce, good choice." I must say it made me chuckle, he was so opinionated about my lunch.

The story does not end there. I went out to my car and parked right next to my car was a past "Dean Ornish Reversal Program" participant. I knocked on

Bob's window. He rolled it down. I said, "Hey, I just got an egg white sandwich."

Bob said he was heading in to do the same. He said that he just got back from Germany. His son lives there. They were celebrating the birth of a new grandson. As any great grandparent would, Bob had a photo. Adorable!

Bob told me how great he feels since he changed his lifestyle habits. He admitted that he overindulged on his trip. We both agreed that he knows how to get right back on track. He values his health and the choice he learned to make which are helping him maintain quality living.

Bob had a heart attack in 1991, followed by stents and then triple bypass surgery. He has described to our team that, at the point he came into the program, he was "at the end of his rope." Now, 80+ years old, Bob is still working because he has so much energy. He looks and feels great because even if he goes off track once in a while, overall, he knows how to make good choices most of the time.

This "most of the time" philosophy gives you the permission to take ownership of what you eat, how often, and when. Are you willing to take that kind of responsibility? Can you choose what is best for your health and quality living most of the time. When you learn this approach and live by it, there is no guilt.

I have seen many people "morph" into other people by being determined to re-pattern their belief systems, break habitual living, and redefine what really brings satisfaction to their lives. I'm sure that Bob is delighted to still be here to meet his new grandson.

When you take ownership of your life and your choices, admit your worst habits, and remain determined to change, then "most of the time" you, too, will be able to say that you make wise choices for eating well.

Muncher Be Aware

Sometimes I still fail to consider that what I am eating may have hidden calories and extra fat, especially if I'm busy, and if I'm not paying attention. Mindless eating can take over at any time. If you aren't careful it can reflect in your waist measurement and scream at you from your scale.

For example, the other day, I wanted a snack and my taste buds were calling for something a little sweeter. I decided on a small bag of" Swiss mix," which is a trail mix containing raisins, dried pineapple, chocolate and butterscotch chips, unsalted peanuts and M & Ms. I like the varied textures and flavor combinations in this kind of mix. I was sitting at my desk, not hiking, which goes against the original intent of eating "trail mix." That's already one strike against me. (I later took a walk to our central supply room, five flights down from my office, to get some "hiking" in.)

In this case, there can be more danger sitting in the office over eating than tripping over a rock or twig on an outdoor trail. The "trip and fall" comes in "checking out" instead of checking into the nutrition facts of what you are eating. In my case, I was savoring the variety of morsels happy to know that I was getting some iron and fiber with my raisins, and some protein with my nuts. I got about halfway through my 2-ounce bag when it hit me that this one bag may not be one serving…oh how I was hoping that it was. However, looking over the nutrition facts, I discovered the serving size was one ounce, much to my disappointment and alarm. If I had continued, I would have eaten double the recommendation for a healthy serving.

One serving of Swiss mix contains 7 ounces of fat (1.5 saturated fat), and 15 carbs (11 of them sugars). I was gaining the 4 grams of protein and the 4 percent iron and 4 percent vitamin C from what I had already eaten. I took a paper clip and closed off the opening of the bag. That officially made it a snack for another day.

It is good to review the concept of serving sizes. On packaged foods there is a panel with nutrition facts that will tell you the servings in a back or container. Like me, wishing you could close your eyes, you may often peak through one eye squinted at the nutrition label. One interesting note, a portion is the amount of food that you choose to eat for a meal or snack. It can be big or small, you decide. A serving is a measured amount of food or drink based on nutrition facts defined by the FDA.

It turns out that many foods that come as a single portion actually contain multiple servings. So "muncher, beware" – or should I say "muncher be aware." It is the unconscious mode of eating that can really sneak in those extra calories that would require lot of extra movement and vigorous exercise to create the balance for over-eating. You may be jolted by the reminder that serving sizes of common foods consist of the following: one slice of bread, one-half cup of rice or pasta cooked, one small piece of fruit, one wedge of melon, one cup of milk or yogurt, 2 ounces of cheese, 2 to 3 ounces of meat, poultry or fish (the size of a deck of cards).

The National Institute of Health (NIH) calls eating larger amounts of food "portion distortion" and says that this eating style is very prevalent compared to years past. "Average portion sizes have grown so much over the past 20 years that sometimes the plate arrives and there's enough food for two or even three people on it. Growing portion sizes are changing what Americans think of as a "normal" portions at home too," observes the NIH.

The NIH report illustrates how what is available in stores and restaurants varies in great measure from 20 years ago. For example, on average, a 140-calorie 3-inch bagel is now replaced with a 350-calorie 6-inch bagel; a hamburger used to be 333 calories is now larger at 590 calories; and a 6.5 ounce, 82-calorie soft drink is now a super-sized 20 ounce soft drink, 250-calories. Read at:
http://www.nhlbi.nih.gov/health/educational/wecan/eat-right/distortion.

Remember to remember to pay attention to the volume and serving sizes you eat. For it has been duly noted that you can't out-exercise a bad diet.

Bounce to Your Best

Are you looking for something that can firm your arms, improve your balance, reduce your body fat, stimulate your lymphatic system, benefit your joints and give you an aerobic workout? It's not too good to be true, it's the positive affect of a rebounder, which is a mini trampoline.

Exercise is a combination of movement and resistance, and a rebounder adds the benefit of G-force to really amp the impact of movement. When you bounce on a rebounder you work against gravitational pressure, resisting the Earth's pull. Alternating weightlessness and double gravity dynamic produced by bouncing forces oxygen into cells. Just 20 minutes on the rebounder is equal to running one hour.

With careful, regular rebounding you can revitalize your body and impact your physical and mental wellness. If you are not a fan of cardio workouts you may be surprised at how much this simple, non-invasive tool can make a potent difference without too much sweat.

"The gentle and constant up-and-down motion helps release an enzyme in your muscle cells that is responsible for splitting open fat cells and converting their contents into energy," says Heidi L. George, breakingmuscle.com.

Rebounding not only uses up stores of fat, it removes toxins by stimulating and toning the lymphatic system. The G-force mentioned earlier strengthens the heart and the musculoskeletal system, establishes better equilibrium, increases capacity for respiration, and protects joints from the impact of exercising on hard surfaces.

Yes, just by bouncing daily you can improve digestion, instigate regular bowel movements (reducing constipation), regulate blood pressure, and benefit the body's immune system. There is a natural increase for fighting disease and irradiating cancer cells by eliminating antigens. Bouncing today can eliminate illness tomorrow.

Besides all of the health benefits rebounding improves your resting metabolic rate. Therefore, more calories are burned for hours after bouncing. Are you hooked yet? Well consider that rebounding affects core muscles and large muscle groups by triggering contraction, resulting in the rhythmic compression of the veins and arteries. This action improves circulation, returning pooling blood back to the heart. The body responds to all of the positive effects of rebounding with deeper relaxation and easier sleep, and has been shown to slow down the aging process

If you are just getting back into an exercise routine, plan on starting slow and steady. Rebounding offers relief from back pain or stiff neck that can result from starting back to exercise after being sedentary. Rebound exercise has been shown to benefit body alignment and posture.

Experts advise to increase your rebounding time gradually. Adults can start with 5 minutes of rebounding and increase their time as their fitness level improves. Seniors can start with 2 minutes several times per day, with at least 30 minutes between rebounding sessions. It's necessary for older people to start gradually in order to give the connective tissue holding the internal organs in place time to strengthen.

If you are new to exercise, have been sedentary or unwell lately or are very overweight, consult your physician before you start a new exercise routine, especially a rebounder workout.

Building Steam

The best way to set direction is by finding the energy to churn the engine of your aspirations. That steam, when you are intending to start a new project, lose weight, or improve your health comes first from within. It is your desire and your drive to succeed that fuels your own engine.

Sometimes we can feel like you're back at the starting block. That is the time to use hope and inspiration to stoke your inner fires. Thinking fresh is a good way to get behind your ambitions and succeed. Set your sights on the horizon of feeling better and celebrating the prize of success.

When I think of stoking inner engines and building adequate steam, I'm reminded of the movie, "Titanic" which so vividly detailed a clear education about what happens when all of the grandeur moving full steam ahead, but without enough foresight, collides with the iceberg. Often when setting new goals, resistance is that iceberg. If you don't have big enough propellers and purposely install an inadequate amount of lifeboats, even with all of the glitz, you're going down.

So begin your fresh new start by clearly deciding how you will fuel your vision and resource your inner steam wisely. The steam engine in its day was a symbol of power. Force and speed can be a boon to aid your direction. It can also be the undoing of the journey leading to wreckage if you don't set out with a clear vision and focus.

Certainty of what you will accomplish, along with determination, will help you steer your ship. Activating the right parameters to guide your project helps you to take the helm and navigate through choppy waters at times. Name specifics of what you want to accomplish. Remaining too general can sink the ship. Deciding to lose 2 pounds a week, making each choice to meet the goal, is far better than knowing you need to lose 30 pounds.

Making sure that you have an enough "life boats" will set up a strong back up plan. Be sure to surround yourself with support from family members, friends, and perhaps professionals if necessary, you strengthen the force of your chosen direction and carve the path with concentrated effort for the biggest result.

Blowing off steam can bring in new vigor. Get to the gym, take a brisk walk at a shopping mall or local school, or complain about your frustrations to a spouse or friend with determination to stay on track. It's ok to be angry and frustrated, but manage it, don't get stuck.

It's no fun being stuck in the doldrums. While it's natural at times to run out of steam, remember that getting stuck is only useful if you admit that you've lost momentum and call on one of your established life boats to press onward and gather new strength.

Gather steam by refocusing on the "why" behind your decision to make a change. You knew you needed something new. "Different" takes a while to own. Recalling your goals and the deeper benefit behind what you intend to achieve is the best way to re-fuel your engine.

As you pick up steam and create momentum your new ideas and choices become habits. These new patterns will become your new way of life. Then, it's full steam ahead as you'll begin to look behind you at the territory you covered to earn the quality of living you target in whatever form you are setting up as new resolutions now.

The honesty of accepting that it is only under your own steam that you will accomplish what you are beginning will help you from the outset to claim victory in the weeks and months ahead.

Whether you feel lost at sea or you're looking for the right road – by land or by sea, knowing clearly what you want to accomplish sets up effective guard rails to make sure you draw a map to meet your objectives.

Dance

All research points to lifestyle as the most significant impact you can have on your triglycerides. Medication can help. Therefore follow your doctor's prescription. However, healthy lifestyle choices are the key to your success in making a difference in your triglyceride count, even more so than other lipids.

Triglycerides provide your body with energy by storing unused calories. Since, like other fats such as cholesterol, they can't be dissolved in blood, triglycerides just float around in your bloodstream. The problem is that too much of both of these fats circulating in the blood can contribute to thickening of the artery walls and hardening of the arteries. This puts you at higher risk for heart disease, stroke and heart attack.

According to the U.S. National Cholesterol Education Program, the guidelines for interpreting triglyceride levels are as follows: Normal, <150; Borderline to high, 150-199; High, 200-499; Very High, $\geq$500.

The good news is that here is clinical evidence that triglycerides respond well, and quickly, to lifestyle changes. The America Heart Association (AHA) suggests the following lifestyle changes to target lowering or maintaining health triglyceride levels:

- **Lose weight.** If you're overweight, losing 5 to 10 pounds can help lower your triglycerides. Motivate yourself by focusing on the benefits of losing weight, such as more energy and improved health.

- **Cut back on calories.** Remember that extra calories are converted to triglycerides and stored as fat. Reducing your calories will reduce triglycerides.

- **Avoid sugary and refined foods.** Simple carbohydrates, such as sugar and foods made with white flour, can increase triglycerides.

- **Limit the cholesterol in your diet.** Aim for no more than 300 milligrams (mg) of cholesterol a day — or less than 200 mg if you have heart disease. Avoid the most concentrated sources of cholesterol, including meats high in saturated fat, egg yolks and whole milk products.

- **Choose healthier fats.** Trade saturated fat found in meats for healthier monounsaturated fat found in plants, such as olive, peanut and canola oils. Substitute fish high in omega-3 fatty acids — such as mackerel and salmon — for red meat.

- **Eliminate trans fat.** Trans fat can be found in some fried foods and commercial baked products, such as cookies, crackers and snack cakes. But don't rely on packages that label their foods as free of trans fat. In the United States, if a food contains less than 0.5 grams of trans fat a serving, it can be labeled trans fat-free. Even though those amounts seem small, they can add up quickly if you eat a lot of foods containing small amounts of trans fat. Instead, read the ingredients list.

You can tell that a food has trans fat in it if it contains partially hydrogenated oil.

- **Limit how much alcohol you drink.** Alcohol is high in calories and sugar and has a particularly potent effect on triglycerides. Even small amounts of alcohol can raise triglyceride levels.
- **Exercise regularly.** Aim for at least 30 minutes of physical activity on most or all days of the week. Regular exercise can boost "good" cholesterol while lowering "bad" cholesterol and triglycerides. Take a brisk daily walk, swim laps or join an exercise group. If you don't have time to exercise for 30 minutes, try squeezing it in 10 minutes at a time. Take a short walk, climb the stairs at work, or try some sit-ups or pushups as you watch television.

The AHA notes that it's also important to control diabetes and high blood pressure if you have high triglycerides and one of these conditions. During "Heart Month," February is a great time to take a look at your triglyceride levels and begin to look forward to making positive changes that can really impact your well-being.

Here's an adage to live by: Life may not always be the party you hoped for, but while you're here you can still choose to dance. With this philosophy, you will lower your triglycerides, and continue to get the exercise you need to maintain healthy levels.

Develop Your Habitable Zone

What do Walt Disney, Arnold Schwarzenegger, and Goldilocks and the three bears have in common? They all know the power of creating the right conditions for success.

First, Walt Disney, a true visionary, said, "Times and conditions change so rapidly that we must keep our aim constantly focused on the future." When creating what you want in your life, training yourself to focus like a laser is necessary. It may take time for all of the right conditions to culminate to achieve the full result you desire. It takes tenacity and goal setting to make the difference and go the distance, outlasting old patterns and challenging unforeseen circumstances.

Next, it is important to know your weaknesses and be prepared to manage them if you are going to succeed. Understanding the importance of establishing committed and set times for conditioning, Arnold Schwarzenegger said, "Training gives us an outlet for suppressed energies created by stress and thus tones the spirit just as exercise conditions the body." How do you "tone the spirit" to stay true to your vision and to meet your goals? To achieve any success, health-wise or otherwise, walking, running, swimming, tennis, bowling, yoga, weight lifting, and aerobics classes are just some of the activities that condition the body and the mind by emphasizing a positive outlet. Choosing your training sets the tone to perceive yourself as a winner. Therefore, you are ready and in-shape when challenges arise. Don't let your true vision fall to the self-sabotage of not taking good care of yourself. Balancing fun and workout is the recipe for a winning attitude. Also, don't underestimate the power of contemplation and prayer.

When astronomers consider whether the right conditions could exist for life on other planets they consider what they call the "Habitable zone." They review if there is any other evidence beyond the atmosphere that might indicate if a planet is capable of supporting life. Additional requirements that measure if a star can "host" a planet, according to Wikipedia, include: Will the star survive long enough for its planets to develop life, and do the planets exist in a region that is the proper distance from the star for that planet (or its moons) to have water remain liquid (that is, not too cold or too hot).

This is also referred to as, "The Goldilocks principle" or "Goldilocks effect" taken from the children's story of Goldilocks and the Three Bears, and refers to the limits required to sustain life on a planet – at least, life as we know it. All conditions must be in perfect combination, "not too hot, not too cold, but just right." Are the right conditions present to sustain water, is there enough heat, but not too much heat. Everything has to be just right.

Are you using Disney's vision, Schwarzenegger's conditioning, and the Goldilocks principle to make everything just right for your success? Do you measure the right conditions to get the result you intend? Do you give your project or intention enough time, thought, practice? Do you set up your environment for success? Do you surround yourself with the right people to get the support you need?

Often times, whether we want change or we are avoiding change, we get stuck in an "inhabitable zone" of our own making, and we're miserable. It's a good habit to regularly measure to determine if how you are currently living is feeding you the right conditions you need to cross the bridge from where you are to where you want to go. Change what does not.

It is important to sharpen your decision-making skills and be sure to scrutinize each choice of action, each thought, and each emotion to create the inner and outer recipe to positively develop your habitable zone. Only you can best decide which conditions keep your dream alive and fuel your outcome through to fruition. It takes careful planning and nurturing, and experimenting with the right conditions to meet your goals and to know the victory of success.

Enjoy Your Road to Success

To achieve true success, quest for people, places and things that really honor your own integrity, and remember to have fun. If you indulge in activities regularly that are counter to your intentions you may feel more disappointment than delight. If you surround yourself with people that dishearten you, your upset can easily lead to frustration and thwart your larger goals, killing your positive outcomes.

Motivational speaker, Dale Carnegie observed that people rarely succeed unless they have fun in what they are doing. That's my message today. Have fun with anything that you are attempting because, according to the experts, and my own experience, when you are enjoying yourself you are more likely to succeed.

"It boils down to looking at everything we do as a process and that each process has steps. If we look at the steps, there is great potential for improvement and fun," says Ron Culberson, author of, *Do It Well. Make It Fun.* Culberson reviews how to make your job more enjoyable, and how to get good at something in a Forbes Magazine interview, www.forbes.com.

For many, it is about giving yourself permission to let go of rigid mindsets and ditch the attitude that you may be attempting to conform to in order to triumph. Yes, work may be involved. However, admonishing yourself with, "I must not eat junk food" will not bring a healthy sense of joy about your goal. When you make your goal a burden, or if you feel overwhelmed, you create a negative push that can stop you from attaining your dreams.

Follow the advice of Michael Jordan, "Just play. Have fun. Enjoy the game." When you put pressure on yourself – imagine how much pressure Michael Jordan must have put on himself, without any fun, you are digging your own proverbial hole. The trick in having fun is to create the right attitude, with the right people to get the best results you can achieve.

Another sports legend, Joe Namath, advised, "When you have confidence, you can have a lot of fun. And when you have fun, you can do amazing things." Thanks Joe, for giving us a clue. Confidence will help you to relax. When gaining a winning attitude knowing you can, even if you are still in practice mode, will lead you to larger and larger achievements.

Building the momentum and confidence to meet your goals also includes support from others. Sometimes life's education, known as trial and error, is a companion to pursuing your ambitions. So be willing to laugh. Laugh at yourself. Laugh with others who are also committed to enjoying life as much as succeeding.

Perhaps it seems counterintuitive to create merriment in pursuit of what you intend to accomplish. I have a dear friend who highly despises what she calls "forced merriment." The kind of life-engaging interest

I am suggesting is genuine (not forced) and targets experiencing the journey, which deepens and enriches winning the prize.

When you include gathering wisdom through joy on the path, there can be no penalty. Honest experience and keeping your aspirations light hearted create the foundation to go well beyond your expectations. Walt Disney said, "It's kind of fun to do the impossible."

Ultimately, it is life philosophy that will determine how much success you have and to what depth you measure your successes. If you create division between meeting your goals and your joy of living, what is the point?

It should be noted, however, that humor or fun without excellence can actually work against you because the credibility is not there, according to Culberson. He suggests doing a good job and having fun. This is a winning combination to celebrate your successes. Take daily inspiration from Dr. Seuss who quipped, "Today was good. Today was fun. Tomorrow is another one."

Fast Food

Sometimes stepping outside of the box can change the view. If you reframe the idea of "fast food" to regard homemade fresh food prepared well, yet quickly, you can benefit from a modernized and healthier view of fast food. You may have to let go of the idea of convenience to steer your health in the direction of nutrition and away from sugar, salt and fat in your diet.

Convenience has won our lifestyles because our fast-paced lives have set us up to yearn for and value ease. Comfort and the service that comes with the fast food concept has perpetuated a health decline in our culture. At times we all feel the need to balance the stress and exhaustion that can pressure even the most mindful eater. Some days we defer to the easiest choice, especially when hunger calls.

We have two options. Either re-frame our view of fast food to include simple and fresh meals at home, or demand more from our restaurants to deliver better, fresher and more nutritious food.

I am calling you to re-evaluate the pace of your life and expectation of what you owe to yourself. We are inundated with the messages that fast paced living delivers convenient flavor-packed eating. People have asked me how to transition out of the loads of salt, fat and sugar, that does not meet the health goals, even if it's the path ease and immediate gratification.

It starts with maneuvering away from convenience and changing what fast food means. When time is still a factor in choice making, steering away from an empty choice, nutritionally speaking, to an active and creative process can bring you and your family delicious, fast, whole and healthy food. One 20-minute shopping trip per week focused mostly on the produce aisle will put fresh fast foods within your reach quickly.

The trap of conventional fast food is often the lack of planning ahead. A perception of the lack of time, plus the reality of the lack of food availability (if you're not a planner) reduces healthy choice options when you are living life "on the run." Even if you are busy, choose better for yourself. Limit eat-outs only to restaurants that serve fresh food. Let's wake up to the importance of ingesting foods that are handled and cooked well. It makes a difference. As individuals, each time we make the choice for ourselves and for our families to expect more in what we are willing to call food, we become leaders of change for the whole culture.

We have to unchain our old thinking from the fast food mentality in order to discover that we can still have the option of relatively fast food right at home, and that it can be healthy and taste good. Expand your definition of fast by incorporating veggie-based meals in your weekly menu plan. I'm not suggesting that you become vegetarian. However, eliminating meat-focused meals twice per week can help speed up how fast dinner is served right at home...in a matter of minutes, with just a little pre-planning. Including eggs or plant-based protein, such as canned black beans or hummus, can get dinner on the table in a jiffy. Less cooking time, yet delivery of speed and flavor.

Gauging our meal choices on convenience alone locks us into a limited living style and can become a void of nutrients that truly feed the body. Remember, you don't have to see the whole staircase, just the first step. Plan a trip to the grocery store and take that first step toward simple, fresh, nutritious home-cooked meals.

Also, make those eating-out decisions while keeping your health as the highest priority. Choose fresh, grilled, steamed, broiled, or baked when eating in or out. Your energy level will increase. Your physical pain will decrease. Your nerves will feel calmer. You'll sleep better. Your overall health will reflect that you've stepped out of the box, changed your pace and your point of view. You can make "fast" a calmer, healthier and happier state of being.

Fat Food

I recently heard someone remark, "Whoever snuck the 'S' in fast food is a clever person." All reports report that the "fast" of fast food living is the real culprit behind the resulting fat that is plaguing our nation. Convenience that includes fat and salt must go.

Research from the Center For Disease Control (CDC) suggests that percentage of calories consumed from fast food is greater by those who struggle with their weight. "Among adults, the percentage of calories consumed from fast food varied by weight status. The percentage of total daily calories from fast food increased as weight status increased. For each age group, obese adults consumed the highest percentage of their calories from fast food."

Researchers found that eating more than twice per week at fast food restaurants is linked to significantly more weight gain over time than occasional visits. Whether you do indulge in fast food regularly or occasionally it may be wise to look up your favorite choices on www.fastfoodnutrition.org. You may be surprised at what you find on this website of fast food nutrition facts. The education may sway you to look elsewhere, like home, for a good meal.

The choice to eat in allows better control of the ingredients you put into what you cook. It is the number one advantage over eating out, followed by portion sizes. There is nutritional value in monitoring the amount of salt and the kinds of fat that are in your meals. With awareness you are less likely to "super-size" your portions.

I have noticed that when I mention the food network, I am not alone in watching the creative process of cooking and the ideas that are inspired when it comes to making great looking and great tasting food. It starts with this kind of inspiration to change our attitudes about what actually counts as food, in both flavor and nutrition.

And it may also lead to a re-valuation of the pace and expectation of what we owe to ourselves as a culture and the health of our families and our bodies. I know it seems crazy that the guest chefs on the television show "chopped" can whip up an entree in 30 minutes. However, I have found that when I have fresh ingredients on hand, I can often make a beautiful and great tasting meal in 30 minutes or less. I can make a pita packed with stir-fry in 15.

The key is to have ingredients on hand to simply preparation of home-cooked meals when you are busy. We have to unchain our thinking from the fast food mentality in order to discover that we can still have relatively fast food, and that it can be healthy.

"I think America's food culture is embedded in fast-food culture. And the real question that we have is: How are we going to teach slow-food values in a fast-food world? Of course, it's very, very difficult to do, especially when children have grown up eating fast food and the values that go with that," comments Alice Waters, one of the most well-known food activists in the United States and around the world.

Waters is an advocate for developing environments that teach and encourage change in American eating habits, such as her creation of the Edible Schoolyard Program, piloted in Berkley, California. Waters serves as a public policy advocate on the national level for school lunch reform and universal access to healthy, organic foods, and the impact of her organic and healthy food revolution.

Eric Schlosser, author of Fast Food Nations says, "Future historians, I hope, will consider the American fast food industry a relic of the twentieth century--a set of attitudes, systems, and beliefs that emerged from postwar southern California, that embodied its limitless faith in technology, that quickly spread across the globe, flourished briefly, and then receded, once its true costs became clear and its thinking became obsolete."

You Are the Solution

I want to share a beautiful quote by Christian D. Larson to offer you a tool to remind you that you can cope with whatever life is giving you. "Believe in yourself and all that you are. Know that there is something inside you that is greater than any obstacle."

I've had many people ask me if there is a solution to stress. I've always answered in the affirmative. It comes first from within. Stress management has an instinctual component. That doesn't mean that we don't rely on outside assistance in any and all ways possible. But I remind people that we have often untapped resources inside of us that we may forget is the best fuel for coping.

"Problem-solving is a natural human talent. We're born solving problems from our first attempts as babies to grasp and crawl. We may not count the thousands of choices we make each day as problem-solving, but that's what they are. So when you focus on solving more complicated problems, have the confidence of knowing that you've got plenty of experience behind you," says the Mayo Clinic staff.

So take heart. Isn't it great to know that you've been an amazing problem solver all along? Many studies about stress and its effects on both the human body and the human psyche, point to teaching stress management as a "treatment" for stress and many related conditions.

We all can learn to identify signs of stress. Acute stress is short term and is tied into our fight or flight response. The symptoms don't cause long-term damage and may include irritability, anger, muscle spasms, tension headaches, racing heart, flatulence, and heartburn.

Chronic stress on the other hand damages our bodies over time with on-going internal or external conditions causing a breakdown of body systems due to the unrelenting stress response being constantly stimulated in the body, leading to coronary artery disease, diabetes, even cancer.

"Chronic stress destroys bodies, minds and lives. It wreaks havoc through long-term attrition. It's the stress of poverty, of dysfunctional families, of being trapped in an unhappy marriage or in a despised job or career," according to an article by the American Psychological Association. This is why building awareness and recovering natural coping skills is essential.

Episodic stress refers to conditions such as if you or someone you know is always in a rush, yet always seems to be late and has too much on his/her plate all of the time. This appears to be an addiction to acute stress, which may lead to hypertension, migraines, angina and heart disease.

All of these stress patterns can be addressed with the practice of stress management, although some conditions will require your doctor and other professionals to bring your body and mind back into balance. Believe in yourself and using your own will to want to begin to take back control of your life patterns is the key to managing and recovering from stress.

Awareness and understanding are the first steps. Knowing what your triggers are, or becoming honest about the circumstances creating internal or external pressure in your life requires reflection. Take the time to stop and look at your life. By identifying stressors you can create strategies to manage them without judgment or blame. Humans were all built for this remember? It's a talent.

New choices are a natural part of adapting and strategizing change. Once you become clear determine if you've seen this pattern before. Remember a time where you found a solution. Maybe this situation requires finding a fresh answer for change. Be open to ask family members or friends you trust for advice or help in seeking a solution. Or seek professional advice from your doctor or counselor.

T.S. Eliot said, "If you aren't in over your head, how do you know how tall you are?" With practice you can measure where you stand in your own life and develop confidence, the support, and the tools to live well. You've made it from birth this far. You are the solution.

Getting in Touch

One of the great mindfulness teachers of our day, Thich Nhat Hanh said, "If you truly get in touch with a piece of carrot, you get in touch with the soil, the rain, the sunshine. You get in touch with Mother Earth and eating in such a way, you feel in touch with true life, your roots, and that is meditation. If we chew every morsel of our food in that way we become grateful and when you are grateful, you are happy."

Because we've all been born with a full set of emotions, pain and suffering can be as prevalent as peace, love and joy. We tend to want to push away sadness, anger, illness. We tend to grasp for and form attachments to what we perceive brings us happiness. Meditation helps that human dynamic to find balance so there's not too much aversion and not too much grasping. We gain a greater understanding that in life there is some challenge, some pain, some suffering, some enjoyment, some happiness, some reward.

Meditation sinks you deeper into your own unique dynamic of thoughts and feelings. As you stop trying to avert what you don't want, and accept life's complexities, you gain the blessings of wisdom, unbound intelligence, true happiness and love. There is a great peace that you live from when you touch into those rewarding qualities. Meditation helps you do that.

Breathing is central to meditation training. Using the rhythm of breath is a wonderful focus in training the mind to be calm and concentrated. Think of meditation as a concentrated form of concentration. When you begin to feel the benefit of just a few minutes of focusing and centering, you won't want to live a day without it. Just as you wouldn't leave the house without taking a shower, you won't want to start the day without at least 10 minutes of sacred practice – whether it be prayer, meditation, inspirational reading. Why call it sacred practice? Because a reverence emerges from within an individual who cultivates self-caring and self inquiry. It makes you humble. It is said that a humble person walks in a friendly world. He or she sees friends everywhere he or she looks, wherever he or she goes, whomever he or she meets. His or her perception goes beyond the shell of appearance and into essence.

All of these practices create an inward dynamic that prepares the practitioner to have a new relationship with the mind and the emotions. Daily preparation to include the sacred inspires us to be more observant, less judgmental, more forgiving, less selfish, more self-assured.

Willingness to take just the few minutes of quiet inner reflection makes more likelihood to put into practice the choice to appreciate all the nuances of living as a caring human, grateful for eating the carrot, or making a difference for someone, or recognizing the difference that is afforded to you by the next person who lends you a hand.

Quiet contemplation and meditation are vehicles to better health. You can think of meditation as a car that you get into and drive inward. It is a practice that becomes easier. As you get comfortable, you know the way.

Developing awareness can affect what you choose to eat and the portion size. Awareness keeps an internal link to what your body is asking. Thirst, the need to get up and take a walk, sleep, are all translated and activated easier when you are in sync with your body. Meditation keeps you in sync.

It has also been clinically proven that meditation positively affects the brain. By rule of thumb, any process that changes your perception changes your brainwaves. Over the long term, meditation trains your brainwaves into balance.

The willingness to connect to your inner dynamic will help you connect to the proverbial carrot and all the life connected to the carrot. When you relax, you open. When you open you expand your viewpoint of the world. In that way, you become grateful and when you are grateful, you are genuinely happy.

Good Vibrations

When you're up against something challenging wisdom may tell you, "This too shall pass." This wisdom in those moments when you are craving something you know you shouldn't eat may prove false. If you are like me…it usually doesn't pass all that easily.

What do you crave? Is there something or someone inside of you calling for a snickers bar, potato chips, cake or pie? Who is that voice? Where is it coming from? It fells real, even though you are sure the real "you" is the voice with the healthy goals.

Research finds that areas of the brain that are responsible for remembering and sensing pleasure are partially behind those callings that we call cravings. And it turns out that, no matter what you are craving, it's often a combination of fat and carbs.

The top foods that people report craving are potato chips, French fries, chocolate, rich ice cream, chocolate chip cookies and macaroni and cheese, according to WebMD.com Do any of these foods ring your bell?

Emotional triggers can also lead you to foods that contain fat, sugar or both.

Stress is also a contributing factor. If you are stressed, it is likely that you may need to create more balance to ensure that you are experiencing enough enjoyment from other sources besides sugary, fat-based foods.

Friendship, the passion of a hobby or other interests, love, a fulfilling career, or developing a stronger sense of belonging deliver forms of nourishment which feed us well-being and satisfaction. Take a look at these areas of your life and be willing to self-assess. What quadrant of your life are you willing to place more attention on? The answer may help you grow in ways other than your waist size.

A physiological reason why you may feel cravings includes dehydration, which mimics feeling hungry. Therefore, drink a glass of water and wait before indulging.

Nutritional deficiencies will also send a message that can feel like cravings, and without proper translation by yourself or professional nutrition counseling may be leading you to fill up with empty calories, leaving your body continuing to feel deprived of life-sustaining nutrients and vitamins that fuel healthy cell reproduction.

The Beach Boys song "Good Vibrations," can be an inspiration towards shifting out of cravings and into gaining the strength of your own focus on balanced living. "Good, good, good, good vibrations" are all around if you tune into the supportive to help you can receive. Positive options create good vibes.

One of my yoga students said that she feels such good vibes in yoga class. Where do you find your good vibes? Knowing the environments, activities and people that uplift and inspire you is essential to busting cravings and staying true to your goals.

Vibration can be thought of as the note you resonate with on your personal piano. When the note is sounded you can tune into that "sound" and feel better. That positive note is the link aligning you with good vibes in your own life. You know the people around you that have good vibes and the ones that have bad vibes.

The "nay" sayers and the troublemakers don't really offer the kind of energy that can uplift and support you and your goals. The next time you are feeling that internal twitch to eat or drink high sugar or fat-laden foods rely on your good vibe resources. If you know a 15-minute walk helps you feel better, or you make a phone call and laugh with a good friend, you are more likely to align with the positive voice and over-ride that craving.

Occasionally, I still give in. If you give in to your craving, enjoy the choice. You can let go of the guilt when you "keep those lovin' good vibrations A'happenin."

The Voice

When I got to the register at work the other day to pay for my lunch (a tuna sandwich on wheat and Brussels sprouts), I told the cashier that I was so proud of myself because I had managed to successfully to over-ride the urge for a coke which led to an over-ride for a diet-coke, which led to an over-ride for a bottled green iced tea. I ended up drinking a hot herbal tea at my desk, nothing added. It was a lot of work as I kept the steady climb toward the better choice.

The cashier agreed that she also has a little voice inside and sometimes it's easier to listen to it. Sometimes it is easier give in and eat or drink those high calorie items. I try to reserve agreeing to the demands of "the voice," which as you know is sometimes a nag, when I am with family and friends. I decide to give in and have that extra piece of pizza or share a piece of cake or pie. But I really do my best to try to stick to over-ride mode when I am eating a regular, mundane breakfast, lunch or dinner. Try it, and see how it works for you. If you don't have one, you may want to install one.

It's important not to give the voice too much power. But as the cashier said, it can be very easy to give in when it is so cold outside and we are bracing against the elements. When cold weather challenges our sensibilities, it's better to reach for something hot, either in temperature or spicy in taste.

Heat increases the sensation of being warm. I like the warmth of ginger. Fresh, in tea or natural ginger candies found at the health food store are great for warmth and they help with digestion. Ginger, or any herbal tea, will keep you hydrated during winter when cold weather robs us of moisture. Hot cider is also good and counts as daily water intake.

Coffee is ok for some hydration but doesn't count toward your daily water intake. The caffeine is the culprit. Keep homemade soups and stews on hand. They will usually contain less sodium and you can add lots of veggies. Cooking or baking healthy recipes at home if you have time warms the house, which balances the cold weather for a home-felt hug.

When the calling for carbs surfaces, do your best to go for complex carbohydrates such as whole grain breads and pastas. When the habit of reaching for cake or cookies becomes a prevalent choice in the winter, it's time to consider whether you may be suffering from "winter depression" called S.A.D. or seasonal affective disorder. This can be triggered by a lack of sunlight in cold weather climates.

When you can name the culprit, you can take your power back. Whole oats with a little brown sugar and cinnamon, low fat brown rice pudding, and legumes and beans, found in lentil soup or turkey chili, are other choices to satiate that craving for carbs that will pack in nutrients, instead of packing on pounds, until the sun returns us to happier, warmer weather.

To understand the body's physiology in the winter, consider that a layer of fat on your body acts as insulation to protect you from the cold. More importantly, your body uses fats to facilitate the absorption of vitamins A, E, K and D. Vitamin D deficiency, can contribute to depression and damage your health. Sunlight, which can be scarce in the winter, aids in vitamin D absorption, and most individuals get less sun when temperatures drop.

Try to include healthy fats in your diet such as fish, nuts, nut butters, olives, avocados and tofu. Keep red meat consumption (one serving is 3 ounces) limited to three times weekly.

Keep reminding that little voice that even thought the body is demanding more calories they don't have to be empty calories. Junk food is persuasive. That is why it takes awareness and the ability to over-ride your urges and cravings for fats and sweets to the best of our abilities. Motivational speaker, Peter F. Drucker says, "What you have to do and the way you have to do it is incredibly simple. Whether you are willing to do it, that's another matter."

If you practice over-riding "the voice" until you find the better choice, at least some of the time, you can you keep over-riding the urge for poor choices and climb the ladder of success.

Wishing

They say that expectation is the mother of all frustration. Wait, that doesn't sound right. We are usually speaking of necessity and the mother of invention. I am proposing the necessity for each of us to hold our dreams close, and then set them free by means of magical imagination we call wishing. If you rush to judgment when things aren't going your way, you may be birthing a big goose egg. But if you are willing to play with the art of wishing, you may find your shiny star.

Start by understanding that false expectations can turn into frustration because wanting more from a person or situation than is realistic can become agonizing. It is better to focus on yourself and cultivate your internal, endless resource of hope for what you can and would like to create.

The opportunities for conventional wishing alone are enough to feed your inner-well with hope and magic. There's your birthday of course. I hope you don't waste that opportunity to blow out your candles. Make a wish. You deserve it. Remember as a child you blew the flutter of the soft, fluffy white dandelions going to seed. From memory you can blow those puffs away again, regaining child-like innocence and establishing your summer wish anew. What did you wish for as a child? It could be the hint of what could bring you happiness now.

Look forward to the turkey's wishbone (the larger the bird the stronger the wish), which lends to the holiday magic and tradition in many homes. Make a wish. Wish on an eyelash fallen on a cheek. Then gently blown away. Wish with coins tossed in a fountain, or by urging a ladybug to fly away home.

Wishing gives a new vantage point, stepping above judgment, softening angst when frustration feels like a cement block. Wishing draws out lighter emotions that invite the heart to smile, releasing burden, and in turn also puts a smile on your face. If you can wish, you can rise to a new level that will help you make the choice to confront the stale view and the emotions that frustration breeds. Yes, even though you feel quite stuck, bring a wish into your life to create a magic wind that can set your sails for a new course.

I ask you not to be "an accomplice" to your own frustration by fueling toxic thoughts and emotions. If you are jaded by life's disappointments, it can feel far-fetched to think that blowing out some candles will change your circumstances. Have the courage to light your candles, sing your own song, and make a difference in your well-being.

Classic author, George Eliot said, "It seems to me we can never give up longing and wishing while we are thoroughly alive. There are certain things we feel to be beautiful and good, and we must hunger after them.

Inner life, and your imagination, is where the spark of good lives within you. Inner life and the calling of the heart keeps the vital magic of living alive. Wishing squashes the multiplication of negativity that feeling stuck brings. Wish upon the first star of the evening. You could certainly shift your perspective, and get you some much needed fresh air. Wish for courage, wish for patience, wish for wisdom, along with the special dream you hold. Remember the rhyme, "Star light, star bright, the first star I see tonight, I wish I may, I wish I might, have the wish I wish tonight."

Grace

I have a friend, I'll call her Grace, who is learning to eat differently, as prescribed by her doctor for her health. She is doing well, and at times can become frustrated. Often, the more conscientious you are with what you do, the more you may struggle when learning new things. You want to do it right.

This is especially true when what you are learning impacts your basic survival instincts, such as what you eat. Give yourself time when creating new habits. Even the most sincere intentions to learn new habits require a margin of trial and error.

In Gracie's case, she is an excellent cook who moves around her kitchen intuitively. She creates excellent meals for her family with ease and perfection because she knows what she likes, and what they like.

I say she is "intuitive" in the kitchen because, as any cook knows, once you've chopped, diced, pureed, minced, sautéd, broiled, baked, fried, roasted, grilled, and steamed enough, you develop your own way of being in the kitchen, and own a familiar relationship with the foods you are used to cooking.

So when your doctor prescribes a diet that cuts out certain foods, or requires you to use new foods that are not part of your usual grocery list, it can feel foreign.

I would call this counter-intuitive. Imagine – you are standing in your kitchen with every intention to use the tofu you just bought. However, you have no idea what to do with it. Even if you have a new recipe, chances are you don't know how to prepare it.

You may ask yourself, "Is it supposed to be this soggy?" And it is still in the shape of the box that it came in…not nearly as appetizing as the rosemary chicken you would normally be cooking.

Likewise, even if you are willing to get more protein and water-soluble fiber from eating beans, the question often is…what do I do with them? How do you make beans interesting? And what do I do with beans the time after that? Especially if they are replacing the Monday night hamburgers….IT DOES NOT COMPUTE!

Grace is a trooper, she is determined to take ownership of the challenge and follow the advice of her Integrative Doctor who is teaching her to change her chemistry through the foods she is eating, in order to protect her health. I admire her courage. It is not easy to find flax and millet bread. It is a specialty item she can't just pick up at the local grocery store. It also takes a special effort to shop for organically grown vegetables.

She is trying out new things slowly and finding her way to new tastes and textures. I don't know if she is playful yet with adding new spices, but she is standing on this new playground with seasonings in hand.

Her goal is to find her way to new "food friends" that she will cherish and love as much as she did the friends in her old lifestyle…she particularly misses creamy textures, cheese sauces, gravies. She will learn how to create a "healthy creamy" – just because that is the kind of person she is, and she values her good health.

Your Will is Your Wheel

Whatever life is calling you to do whether getting back to exercise, solving a problem, or helping a friend, when you choose willingly to be aligned with the task the result will bring you satisfaction. Willingness helps to maintain a sense of equilibrium. A strong will helps to hold a feeling of peaceful calm when doing what life is asking you, even if you don't necessarily "like" it.

Whatever the challenge, know you can amplify your response to what life asking you by being willing to step up. Those very circumstances employ an inner builder that will help forge a better relationship with your inner life, your outer life, and those around you. Imagine giving life all of the characteristics we can aspire to – integrity, goodness, wisdom, power, hope, trust. This "person" is like a mentor who can help develop the intention to listen, to face obstacles and resistance, and to move through challenges.

With this positive perspective you give life the power to help you gather the strength to jump over hurdles and leap through hoops. The advantage of developing "the character" of life conditions you to build amazing qualities in yourself through your experiences.

John Steinbeck said, "A journey is a person in itself; no two are alike. And all plans, safeguards, policing, and coercion are fruitless. We find that after years of struggle that we do not take a trip; a trip takes us."

Life is taking us somewhere. Individually you have the opportunity to experience a personal journey to come to know, revere and respect yourself more, and to build more compassion and empathy for others. Are you drifting along, or focused and on purpose? It's all in where to put your attention.

"You drift through life and let things happen to you, or go by design and say, 'This is what I'm intended to do'," says Rick Warren, author of The Purpose Driven Life. The best way to know what life is asking is to look around you and see what is most needed in your personal life, in your family life, at work and in your community. Where there can be improvement, or you can be of service, is where life is calling you to make a difference.

Making a difference is making life better even though there are highs and lows. Exchange boredom for focus, and turn procrastination into action. In the journey of your life each challenge and every victory gains you your own understanding. Personal understanding becomes the fuel for you to answer life's beckoning.

Some may see change as destructive because going with changes means life doesn't stay the same. Change however is what keeps us fresh and alive. It is the voice of your heart calling to create the best that you have to give and the highest good that you can contribute. Loss is hard. Change can feel impossible. Don't give up on life. Life is that ocean of endless possibilities that brings you blessings, surprises and gifts to celebrate and share.

The Greatest Thank You

In 1839, New York resident, Abner Doubleday, created the game of baseball in his own backyard. The first official baseball game was played in1846; in 1876 the first professional baseball league was formed. The momentum of this American pastime has been building ever since. Each year it is estimated that 21 million hotdogs are consumed at baseball games. I suspect that is a low-ball estimate. If you lined up all of the hotdogs end to end, they would round the bases 29,691 times. Now that's American. If you add the unique ingredient of the singing of the National Anthem to kick-off the game, you have a recipe that feeds our American souls.

"One of the powerful things about music, and a powerful thing about an anthem — it builds community when we sing it together. We have a such a big country, with millions of millions of people, and we know the collective rituals, singing the songs together," said Mark Clague a professor of musicology, the director of research at the University of Michigan, and the founder of the Star-Spangled Music Foundation. He's a big believer in the song's impact on American culture.

I agree that singing our National Anthem at local and professional sporting events is unifying and as powerful as a dedicated moment of silence. I always feel a sense of joint reverence and pride when singing along. The experience delivers an allegiance to the ideals that we, and our country stand for. We are heading into a weekend that is set aside to recognize and honor the most patriotic of all Americans. Memorial Day weekend is upon us, and is our time as a nation to remember our veterans who have fallen. Did you know that in December of 2000, Congress passed a law requiring Americans to pause at 3 p.m. local time on Memorial Day to honor the fallen?

Named "The National Moment of Remembrance" this observance encourages all Americans to pause wherever they are at 3 p.m. local time on Memorial Day for a minute of silence to remember and honor those who have died in service to the nation. As Moment of Remembrance founder Carmella La Spada states: "It's a way we can all help put the memorial back in Memorial Day." http://www.va.gov

Over the years I've proudly attended Memorial Day morning parades and services for our veterans. I have been very touched to see and feel the emotion of those who are survived soldiers. This year, I plan to establish this moment of remembrance observance with my family and friends at 3 p.m. on Memorial Day Monday. I invite you to, also.

While we may all be gathered near our grills or around our picnic tables, or already lulled into our post hot-dog nappy around 3 p.m., let's agree to shift our awareness to the larger meaning behind Memorial Day. We can make this another meaningful American ritual, like singing the National Anthem, dedicated to focus on this special moment of silence in recognition of those who sacrificed so much so that we can kick off our summer with all of the fun and freedoms we enjoy and deserve.

Bob Dylan said, "A hero is someone who understands the responsibility that comes with his freedom." Dying for freedom and justice is the ultimate responsibility. We can all celebrate our heroes and show gratitude if we create a genuine moment of silence in our lives to value their bravery and sacrifice. For a moment we are called to be American contemplatives. This mindful act can impact our culture and our youth to preserve and to shape our story of freedom and justice for all. It is our great honor to especially remember our heroes who have fallen as we to continue discovering the realization of our personal pursuits of happiness.

On May 30, 1868, President Garfield addressed the several thousand people gathered at Arlington National Cemetery. "If silence is ever golden," Garfield said, "it must be beside the graves of 15,000 men, whose lives were more significant than speech, and whose death was a poem the music of which can never be sung."

Your Philosophy
Points Your Direction

Your life philosophy can be your launching pad and your safety net, or your personal perspective may be the hole you are sitting in, dug with self-defeating behaviors and self-sabotage. It's all about what you believe about yourself and life that is steering outcomes. Are you spotlighting or blinding your vision.

I live by the adage, everybody wants happiness, nobody wants pain, but you can't have a rainbow without a little rain. Yes, learning to embrace the good and the bad, the ease and challenge of life enhances your feeling of fulfillment. Do you know what you really think about your relationship with life? Are you willing to learn and grow?

Just spending a little more time contemplating how you want to meet life can deepen your life philosophy because you will gain awareness about what life means to you, what you want to get out of living, and what you want to give back. Introspection gives a point of view and focus to determine how to throw your best pitch and how to best catch those curve balls.

With some regular, quite reflection you begin to understand what and who resonates with your personal goals. You become clear about what you wish to contribute. You sharpen your personal style which becomes your rich way of interacting with yourself, others and life.

What you think about what life offers and stands for is an important matter, and determines your character and the quality of what you share and receive. Your life philosophy is directly related to what you offer and what life offers you. You are the creator of the fabric of what you are living. You spin what you see and what you hear. Examining deeper you study what you feel and what you perceive through your perspective and notions. You can change the trajectory and impact of what happens and what you choose next. This can give new meaning to everything around you.

Weaving your life's tapestry from countless moments of exhausting jabs, if you believe life is a fight is not a commanding philosophy, but a demanding one. The framework you are living in that negative point of view can become heavy and burdensome with a "one-two punch" to the proverbial gut.

You choose what you value by your thoughts, feelings and actions. These components are the philosophical steps on which you move up and/or down the personal staircase of life either creating quality living, or stumbling and falling into autopilot, disappointment, and even despair.

You are the container of your philosophy -- you hold your thoughts, feelings, beliefs and choices within you. What you think and feel about life is what is guiding you now. So if you are not pleased with what is before you, you also can change your mind, your feelings, and your direction.

What is most interesting about life philosophy is that is it built by life experiences. How you choose to translate what happens in your life matters greatly. "It's no use going back to yesterday, because I was a different person then," said Lewis Carroll in Alice in Wonderland.

So the good news is that no matter what has happened and what you've interpreted it to mean, you and I, and everyone are still evolving and each of us has the opportunity to redefine what life means because we are all moving forward. Life is happening and so are we. Picture a world where we all aspire to be better and do better.

Please don't rain on my parade, join in celebrating my rainbow.

II

Yoga: Developing Self-Awareness

Benefits Of Daily Yoga

The benefits of incorporating yoga-based exercises into your daily routine are numerous. Also referred to as "stress management" in our culture, these ancient techniques have a positive impact on all the systems of the body.

Research is showing that when you consistently include gentle stretching and breathing into your daily lifestyle you will lower you blood pressure and improve your circulation, your sleep patterns, and your strength and flexibility.

Gastrointestinal issues improve in both men and women. This is due to the massage that you give to your organs and glands from creating a squeeze and soak affect while deeply breathing.

Cardiovascular disease is greatly improved with increased circulation and increased amounts of oxygen in the body. Another powerful affect is the regulation and slowing of the heart rate and respiratory rate. Cholesterol levels also improve.

Yoga's stretching and breathing helps combat aging through a natural detox process, resulting in the release of toxins and tension. Much of the aging process is due to the breakdown of our skin and tissues from toxins that remain trapped in the body. The physical stretching prepares your body for sitting quietly, which can profoundly impact your mental and emotional well-being, creating an awareness of inner peace.

Gaining peace of mind and improving your mood is another advantage of yoga-based stress management. This is the practice of "you meeting you." It is an inward exploration that many of us, especially men, are not taught to take seriously.

Never being taught, and continuing to not give yourself permission to explore your body and mind patterns, can result in an inability to concentrate, stress, anxiety, depression, or hostility.

Be willing to create some quiet time to relax and breathe. Turn off the television and phones. Make yourself comfortable. Some people use a small blanket around their shoulders to symbolize creating a boundary between the outside world and the time they are taking to go inward.

Then, just be still. Relax and breathe. Close your eyes, or create a soft, relaxed outward gaze. Relax the muscles of the face and jaw. Sometimes this practice can be done without much preparation. However, if you are anxious or hold a lot of tension in your body, you may want to learn the gentle movement and stretching elements of yoga which will help you get more out of your quiet time.

Yoga is all about you. It is non-competitive, focus on what you feel and how it is impacting you. Only you know what you are thinking. Only you can feel your own sensations and emotions. Only you can breathe your breath with more awareness.

To seek instruction to learn the physical poses and stretches, look for a gentle yoga class or a class that is specifically for beginners. You may also feel more comfortable in a "chair yoga" class. Be willing to try more than one class and more than one instructor until you find the right fit.

Core Focus – Good Patterning

Do you look down at your stomach and wonder, where did this flabby mass come from? Weight loss may be on your agenda...but have you also considered the importance of core strengthening?

The muscles around your abdomen, back and pelvis are considered the body's "core." It is the trunk of your body that contributes to the quality of the way you physically balance, walk, and run. It is important to have good muscle tone.

All your movements begin in the core. It can influence the ease or difficulty of how you climb the stairs or lift objects. Your posture, sitting or standing straight, is determined by the strength of your core.

I am an energetic person who gets a lot of movement during the course of a day. I teach several yoga classes in a week, practice yoga at home, and I have a personal walking program. However, I totally avoid traditional core strengthening exercises. You know, the crunches, reverse crunches, oblique cross-over crunches. Uuugh!

That just sounds so awful, mostly because I often feel neck strain if I am not careful when doing these exercises. Whether or not you like crunches, committing to developing good core patterns is essential.

Becoming very aware of the way that you sit and stand is important to maintain the integrity of your posture and your core. This strengthens abs and protects your back.

It is a process of learning to work with gravity, instead of gravity working against you. Since gravity is pulling you downward all of the time, developing a pattern of lifting up through the top of the head will naturally engage the core muscles.

Standing into both of your feet evenly with toes pointing forward is essential for the proper foundation to support good posture. Making a conscious habit of lifting your waist off of your hips. Also the action of "lifting your heart," will help you stand tall and will open the front of your body and engage the back muscles. At first you may feel like a toy soldier, until your back muscles strengthen to your new normal. This happens quickly with regular practice.

If you are sitting, the same awareness of lifting the upper body (the heart upward) will send you deeper into your "seat" and create this important good pattern for lift and strength.

This action of lifting the upper body engages all of the muscles in the trunk, which is the seed of effective core strengthening. Another exercise to include in your routine is called "abdominal bracing." Pull your navel inward toward the spine. Don't hold your breath. Make sure that you can still breathe in and out evenly. This firming of the abs, practiced regularly, will contribute to the goal.

Core strength is also the key to maintaining physical balance. Another way to improve your core is to practice standing on one foot. If you feel unsteady start with a chair in front of you, with the chair back facing towards you. Holding onto the chair back will help you to feel steady.

If using the chair, slowly practice lifting arms out in front of you, returning hands to the chair as necessary for support. Start with 15 or 20 seconds on each foot and work up to one minute on each side.

You may want to consider investing in an exercise ball. It will do similar strengthening for your core. This can be used if you sit a lot at work or at home. Replace your chair with the ball at least 5 to 10 minutes to start. Keep feet on the floor, legs bent, back straight.

Yoga Benefits Everyone

The question, "Which came first the chicken or the egg," is a reference to deadlock situations, a puzzle where the answer creates the problem. In our culture, especially in more conservative communities, this quiz can be applied to yoga class as well.

Do any of you remember the song, "There's a Hole in My Bucket." It starts with a man, Henry, telling his wife, "Dear Liza," that there's a hole in his bucket. After a series of verses in which Liza tells Henry what to do to fix the bucket: get water to sharpen the knife, to cut the straw, to fix the hole. But there's a hole in the bucket.

Women often notice in community yoga classes that there are not many men coming to yoga class. Women align with yoga class intuitively because they feel the benefits immediately due to being more "in tune" with their body. Upper body strengthening, more flexibility and a sense of well-being are just some of the benefits they enjoy, within and without. Many of them voice how much they know their husbands could benefit too.

In our culture, men don't embrace yoga the same way that women do, mainly because many men get the impression yoga is for women. Why? Because, often, there are only women in the yoga classes! There's a hole in the bucket. Gridlock in perception has kept the door closed tight for many men who could be gaining the important benefits that yoga delivers.

Men have the same needs to create blood flow to the heart, kidneys and adrenal glands, and detox the liver, gall bladder, digestive system and spleen. Yoga can be adapted for any age in a variety of levels and ranges. Depending on where you need the stretch, you may hold certain positions longer to allow muscles to lengthen and release toxin build-up.

Held positions allow the body to slowly acclimate to better physical patterning that occurs over time to reduce factors of repetitive motion, tension or over-use of muscles, poor posture and other unhealthy structural misalignments, and sedentary lifestyle. Tension in the muscles not only comes from the demands of life on your physical body. Gravity plays a role in how we maintain balance, flexibility and strength. Gravity is always compacting the joints and the spine. We all need to create patterns to work with gravity, so gravity doesn't work against us.

Yoga works your whole body, enhances your ability to focus and improves sleep patterns. No matter what your gender these are more than perks.

Finding Your Yoga

C'mon inner peace, I haven't got all day...can you admit when you could use a little more inner and outer flexibility, and a little more conditioning to access patience, peace, and calm. There's an old yoga saying, "I bend, so I don't break." That is the concept of yoga practice. You first learn to meet yourself, and that practice helps you meet the world with more strength, more flexibility, more grace.

There is a momentum building in our culture to embrace the good that mindful stretching, bending, strengthening and breathing can contribute to your well-being. The Department of Health & Human Services recognizes the benefits of yoga. The nod toward the practice of yoga concepts is intended to inspire the pubic to embrace a healthy lifestyle and embrace education about healthy patterns yoga can support.

Yoga can improve circulation, balance blood sugars, tone muscles and organs, strengthen bones, and positively condition the nervous system. Yoga is also a stress and pain reliever, and can be instrumental in weight loss because it reduces stress hormones such as adrenaline and cortisol, which keep the body in fight or flight mode, often locking on those stubborn pounds. Yoga practice also develops the habit of mindful eating.

Yoga is different from the motivation and competition of self and other that comes with cardio exercise. It's not an activity as much as it is a state of exploration and learning. It isn't based on whether or not you need to – or want to -- lose weight or any other goal. It doesn't matter if you own special equipment. A yoga mat is optional but can support the habit and commitment of taking time daily to breathe and stretch. Yoga does not try to fix anything or change who or what you are. It reveals and continues to develop your flexibility and strength. Yoga practice also works on the inside. It deepens how patient, understanding, compassionate and peaceful you are toward yourself and others.

The only requirement is the commitment to meet yourself for your own physical, mental and emotional health and well-being. The intention is not to fix or change anything. Yoga practice increases self-awareness and self-acceptance, and diminishes self-criticism and self-judgment.

The wisdom of Confucius says, "What the superior man seeks is in himself; what the small man seeks is in others."

Yoga classes around the country are growing. Both men and women are pursuing the many benefits, which can make a difference in anybody's health. There are many different styles and levels of yoga. Finding the style and instructor that is right for you is worth the search.

With the practice of yoga you learn to tend to your well-being wisely, learning where you can go, surprising yourself that you can evolve and often go farther than you thought you could on your road to health and balance.

Sing a Song

One of the benefits I gained by following a regular yoga practice is that I have become a better singer. I admit that there may be critics who could argue my claim of enhanced song, but I don't see anyone covering their ears.

The regular stretching from yoga improves the flexibility of my shoulders, and front and back of my neck. The regular breathing practice maintains the strength of the diaphragm. Singing a song is like doing several big, long exhales. So the better your lung capacity, the better your crooning will be.

The interesting thing is that studies have shown that singing actually can alleviate stress, decrease your blood pressure, and lower your heart rate. So go ahead, keep singing in the shower – or anywhere else for that matter.

In one study, over a three-year period, a group of singers, ages 55 and over, were followed and examined to see how singing affected their health.

The Seniors Singing Chorale, at the Levine School of Music in Washington D.C., showed "significant health improvements compared to those in the control groups," according to the study.

In the three years, there were 30 fewer doctor visits, fewer eyesight problems, less depression and less need for medication. Participants reported feeling better both in daily life and while singing, and noticed that their voice quality was improved. They also noticed they could breathe easier and had better posture.

Another finding is that using your diaphragm to sing is a good way to promote a healthy lymphatic system, which in turn promotes a healthy immune system. The lymph system keeps toxins moving along. So don't be shy, belt out those show tunes…"When the red, red robin goes bob, bob, bobbin' along" might actually keep the red blood cells prevalent, and the white blood cells ready for strong defense.

By the way, if you are shy, singing will actually bring you out of your shell. Singing can be a confidence booster and is a great release. So if you're stressing, or feeling a little down, you may want to sing the blues. There's a good chance that's why the Blues style of music was created…it just helps you feel better to sing.

Singing develops a different intonation in your voice and puts extra emphasis, such as in crescendo, which can affect your mood differently than when you are talking. You may actually be stirring up the "feel good" hormones just by singing along with the radio.

Singing is also being applied as therapy for people who have been traumatized. Great physical or psychological pain can relieved by blocking a lot of the neural pathways that pain travels through, by singing, according to Dr. Patricia Preston-Roberts, a board-certified music therapist in New York City.

It is a scientific fact that a different area of the brain is used for singing than for speaking. Research is now studying the "feel good" affect of singing for people with Alzheimer's Disease, dementia or memory problems. Initial results indicate that singing does have beneficial effects on cognitive powers, emotions and physical abilities for this population as well.

It's Time For Some Remodeling

How would you like to stop your lower back pain or that recurring stiff neck? How would you like to feel better? Did you ever consider remodeling your back and spine? Is that like remodeling your kitchen…Sort of.

Wait – you say, you don't have back pain…well not yet, anyway. The question is who's got your back? In this case you do. How does it feel?

Statistics predict that almost everyone can suffer from some back pain at some time in their life. Between 60 and 80 percent of the U.S. adult population has low back pain at some point, according to arthritistoday.com.

Acute back pain lasts from a few days to a few weeks and gets better without any treatment. Back pain that lasts more than 3 months is considered chronic, but can usually be treated without surgery.

Let me repeat the old yoga adage, "If you don't hear the whispers, you'll hear the screams." This yoga philosophy applied to back and spine health is equal to Benjamin Franklin's observance, "an ounce of prevention is worth a pound of cure."

In the treatment of back pain when you can take the pressure off of your spine, you make the spine more durable. Strengthening the muscles around the spine can protect your back from injuries and strain. Focus on muscle strength will naturally improve your posture and your core.

"Low back pain is the fifth most common reason for all doctor visits in the United States, with direct health care costs estimated to top $26 billion," according to a joint study by the American College of Physicians and the American Pain Society.

Self-care is indicated when there is no serious underlying condition. Self-care includes stretching your hamstrings, getting enough sleep, focusing on good nutrition to help the healing process. Gain strength and flexibility of the back and spine with therapeutic stretching from yoga or similar modalities. Also consider including meditation to reduce stress.

If you have back pain, give yourself the permission to allow that pain to offer you a time to learn self-care, and an opportunity to build toward a lifetime of health and well-being. This is the time, whether you currently are experiencing back pain or not, to learn and to practice the tools to protect your back and spine.

Doctors, physical therapists, and yoga teachers specializing in back pain are all good resources for you to learn the techniques you will need to create flexibility and strength. Tissue remodeling takes time and patience. Dedicate yourself to supporting the back and spine that supports you. Just like other remodeling projects, it takes time.

Studies have shown that those who practice yoga for as little as twice a week for 8 weeks make significant gains in strength, flexibility, and endurance, which is a basic goal of most rehabilitation programs for back pain or neck pain, according to spine-health.com.

Therapeutic exercises practiced consistently can begin to establish new healthy patterns, and reduce pain. Gentle yoga is best, and safe for everyone. Find a teacher who can adapt stretching to meet your health issue.

Besides learning a back-strengthening stretch routine, pattern yourself to sit and stand up straight, lose weight to reduce the load and strain on your back, stay active, and avoid heavy lifting or lift objects mindfully by remembering to engage your core.

Dwight D. Eisenhower said, "The older I get the more wisdom I find in the ancient rule of taking first things first, a process which often reduces the most complex human problem to a manageable proportion."

Whether or not you are currently experiencing back pain, developing your self-care program in a "manageable proportion" is wise advice. Be willing to take the small steps toward the strengthening of your back and spine. Take action. Preventing back pain is better than treating it!

Say What?
What is Your Posture Saying About You

Your posture is directly related to how you feel in your body. It is also the way you meet the world. Does your posture communicate your confidence, or is your body announcing you are feeling the weight of gravity pulling your down?

Chiropractors, Personal Trainers, Physical Therapists, Massage Therapists and Yoga Teachers can all be considered posture exercise professionals. They can help with pain management. Individualized exercise plans can be very powerful medicine.

As a Certified Yoga Therapist, I have an eye for reading the information someone's body gives me, just by the way they stand and move. Gravity is always pulling down. As a result, if you don't pay attention to the patterns in your body, you may be living with the result of rounded shoulders, weakened muscles and connective tissues. Poor posture is all about losing body integrity.

Therefore, the down-trodden, the lazy and the weak also have a body screaming for more strength and flexibility. Your body may speak your emotions, even if you aren't tuned into them. Depression and other heavy emotions may also show up in the expression of body posture.

Even your digestion and breathing problems may be influenced by poor posture. Ultimately, you will improve your health if you improve your posture. Focusing on strengthening your posture is worth the effort. In as little as two to three weeks, you may feel a significant impact on re-patterning your joints, neck, shoulders and spine. The more you make the correcting patterns part of your daily lifestyle, the more lasting the result. This is how you shape new habits to help you feel well in your body.

Consider that your current patterns are part of your daily lifestyle. If you live without awareness of how you are standing sitting and moving, it could be part of the reason for those headaches, neck cricks and your nagging lower back pain. Your feet, knees, hips and ankles may also be shouting about your poor posture habits.

Improving your posture is an anti-aging decision that can also become a positive decision to help you avoid or repair injury. Body awareness is a key component to correcting your posture. Tai chi, Yoga and Pilates can be great resources for cultivating an intimate knowledge of what is healthy and unhealthy in your stance and posture.

Your seat (when you're sitting) and your feet (when you're standing) are the foundations of your body. It is important to make sure that you sit in a supportive chair and wear supportive shoes. Pay attention to how you hold your body when you drive, speak on the phone, or play video games.

At work, especially, it is wise to start addressing the demanding patterns that may be exhausting your body. Sitting at the computer, having to stand long hours or repetitive motion can negatively impact your body structure.

If you do feel out of alignment or physically stressed, make a decision to develop a new stance for your health and well-being.

Refreshing Laughter

Last week, I was moved to tears by a story about a man and his arthritic dog, Schoep. John Unger and his dog Schoep used to float in Lake Superior, at least 10 minutes each day, if the water temperature permitted, as a form of comfort and therapy for the aging dog.

The on-line photo is priceless, and very touching. It shows the two floating in the water while the dog rests his sleeping head on his owner's chest. See the photo by Googling "Today Pets, floating man with dog." The care and companionship is a torch to the heart. I felt sorrow when I heard that Shoep, despite all of the outpouring of support, died. He lived to be 20 years old! Amazing for any breed.

This got me thinking about how much fun I have with my dog, Jazz. She is a Tibetan terrier. She loves to play "Squirrel." I do the tossing. She does the chasing. The laughter goes both ways...if you're a pet owner; you know when your pet is laughing along with you. There is nothing else like it.

Laughter is important for vibrant health. Laughter relaxes the whole body, releases endorphins (the "feel good hormones"), boosts the immune system, and protects the heart by improving the function of blood vessels and blood flow.

I find that playing with the dog is so rewarding and relaxing. I say that Jazz is a "puppy master, teaching me her puppy ways." If a dog lifestyle doesn't work for you, may I suggest a Guinea pig? Did you know that Guinea pigs chuckle? Or perhaps a cat or a turtle suits you. A pet can at least urge you to smile.

If a pet is absolutely off limits for you, there are other ways to infuse laughter into your life. Seek out fun-loving, funny people. Host a game night with friends. Get silly with children, or watch a funny movie or television show. Any activity that creates laughter leads to improved moods that affect your health.

"The kind of thought we get depends upon the type of hormones circulating in the blood which are released depending upon the state of mind. When one is under fear more negative chemicals are released in the blood resulting in more negative thoughts and feelings," says Dr. Madan Kataria, founder of Laughter Yoga International.

Laughing Yoga has been developed as a brand of stress management that emphasizes the activity of laughing. You can start with smiling while sitting quietly (eyes opened or closed). Then imagine uproarious laughter happening on your insides. Remembering the feeling of laughter has its own effects.

Another Laughing Yoga technique is to place your hand on your heart and begin to laugh out loud, sending the laughter to yourself and others. Just like praying, they don't have to be there. This isn't "forced merriment." It is a simple stringing together of ha-ha-

ha-ha out from the mouth as you intention to send good intentions and blessings to yourself and others.

The founder of the laughing yoga concept is convinced that if we would all begin to focus on daily laughter in this way, we could have world peace.

Alan Alda, the actor, said, "When people are laughing, they're generally not killing each other." Laughter refreshes any relationship and unites people during difficult times. Milton Berle said, "Laughter is an instant vacation."

My advice is to "vacation" often by laughing a lot. All of your cells and all of your systems including your mind, will benefit from engaging in the jovial, the silly and the funny side of life, which brings rewarding and worthwhile health and happiness.

So I'll leave you with a chuckle this week. This is an unknown quote, "Sometimes I laugh so hard the tears run down my leg." On occasion, this is true for me…I hope it's true for you, because it means you are engaged in some very powerful laughter!

I Bend, So I Don't Break

C'mon inner peace, I haven't got all day…are you able to admit when you could use a little more inner and outer flexibility, and a little more conditioning to access patience, peace, and calm. There's an old yoga saying, "I bend, so I don't break." That is the concept of yoga practice. You first learn to meet yourself, and that practice helps you meet the world with more strength, more flexibility, more grace.

There is a momentum building in our culture to embrace the good that mindful stretching, bending, strengthening and breathing can contribute to well-being. The Department of Health & Human Services has officially designated September to be National Yoga Month. The nod toward the practice of yoga concepts is intended to inspire the pubic to embrace a healthy lifestyle and education about health benefits of yoga.

Yoga improves circulation, balances blood sugars, tones muscles and organs, strengthens bones, and positively conditions the nervous system. Yoga is also a stress and pain reliever, and can be instrumental in weight loss because it reduces stress hormones such as adrenaline and cortisol, which keep the body in fight or flight mode, often locking on those stubborn pounds. Yoga practice also develops the habit of mindful eating.

Yoga is different from the motivation and competition of self and other that comes with cardio exercise. It's not an activity as much as it is a state of exploration and learning. It isn't based on whether or not you need to, or want to, loose weight or any other goal. It doesn't matter if you own special equipment, even though using a yoga mat is popular, it is not necessary to show up and breathe and stretch. Yoga does not try to fix anything or change who or what you are. It reveals and continues to develop your flexibility and strength. Yoga practice deepens how patient, understanding, compassionate and peaceful you are toward yourself and others.

The only requirement is the commitment to meet yourself for your own physical, mental and emotional health and well-being. The intention is not to fix or change anything. Yoga practice increases self-awareness and self-acceptance, and diminishes self-criticism and self-judgment. The wisdom of Confucius says, "What the superior man seeks is in himself; what the small man seeks is in others."

Yoga classes around the country and in our own region are growing. Both men and women are pursuing the many benefits, which can make a difference in anybody's health. There are many different styles and levels of yoga. Finding the style and instructor that is right for you is worth the search.

Rather than contending with the riggers of working out (which has its own health benefits), you learn to tend to your well-being wisely, learning where you can go, surprising yourself that you can evolve and often go farther than you thought you could. Consider it an opportunity to discover more about your ability to become the best you you can be.

ABOUT THE AUTHOR

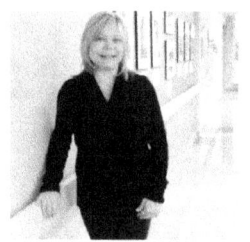 A wellness consultant, educator and promoter of healthy lifestyle concepts and yoga-based therapies for over 20 years, **LORI BROTHERS** has been sharing her perspective about the beautiful practice of yoga and the development of personal awareness for the benefit of health and lifestyle empowerment.

Through her writing, Brothers reveals the personal gift that each life experience offers. A champion for her fellow human beings, she calls them to more deeply value the unique journey of personal perspective, and the power of conscious choice making.

Brothers presents entertaining and heart-felt direction for healthy and well living. She offers encouraging and inspiring upliftment. With a friendly voice Brothers motivates her readers, students and clients to embrace the unique gift of personal experience that each human life unfolds.

A life coach and a counselor of the human spirit, Brothers examples her philosophy of living authentically and leads through sharing lessons for wisdom-based growth. She suggests better-to-best living through educating for greater understanding regarding the power of awareness and the evolution of choice.

A graduate of Youngstown State University with a B.A. in English and Journalism, Brothers is a freelance writer who authors *Healthy Living*, a weekly column for the *New Castle News* in New Castle, Pennsylvania. *The Best of Healthy Living* is a collection of reader favorites.

Brothers is a certified Integrative Yoga instructor and a certified Phoenix Rising Yoga Therapist. As a Stress Management Specialist and later as the Director, Brothers' passion to educate the re-patterning of healthy living led her to deliver the Dean Ornish Program for Reversing Heart Disease: a national research project that is clinically-proven to reverse heart disease and its risk factors. From 2003 through 2014, Brothers facilitated positive life change for heart patients through Jameson Hospital in New Castle, Pennsylvania.

Mother of two adult daughters, Brothers resides in Columbiana, Ohio and currently works as a Public Relations Development Specialist for Jameson Health System. She continues to deliver community yoga classes to students of all walks of life. Through *The Best of Healthy Living*, Brothers is honored to extend the reach of her teachings to improve the lives of others.

www.ingramcontent.com/pod-product-compliance
Lightning Source LLC
Chambersburg PA
CBHW062006280526
45787CB00005B/1996